KU-253-644

OXFORD MEDICAL PUBLICATIONS

THE BOWEL BOOK

BONNYBRIDGE LIBRARY
BRIDGE STREET
BONNYBRIDGE
STIRLINGSHIRE FK4 1AD
TEL. 503295

Oxford University Press makes no representation, express or implied, that the drug dosages in this book are correct. Readers must therefore always check the product information and clinical procedures with the most up to date published product information and data sheets provided by the manufacturers and the most recent codes of conduct and safety regulations. The authors and the publishers do not accept responsibility or legal liability for any errors in the text or for the misuse or misapplication of material in this work.

FALKIRK COUNCIL LIBRARIES

30124 02466219 1

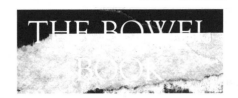

THE BOWEL BOOK

A Self-help Guide for Sufferers

Dr Michael Levitt

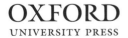

OXFORD
UNIVERSITY PRESS

OXFORD

UNIVERSITY PRESS

Great Clarendon Street, Oxford OX2 6DP

Oxford University Press is a department of the University of Oxford.
It furthers the University's objective of excellence in research,
scholarship, and education by publishing worldwide in

Oxford   New York

Auckland   Bangkok   Buenos Aires   Cape Town   Chennai
Dar es Salaam   Delhi   Hong Kong   Istanbul   Karachi
Kolkata   Kuala Lumpur   Madrid   Melbourne   Mexico City
Mumbai   Nairobi   São Paulo   Shanghai   Singapore
Taipei   Tokyo   Toronto

and an associated company in Berlin

Oxford is a registered trade mark of Oxford University Press
in the UK and in certain other countries

Published in the United States
by Oxford University Press Inc., New York

© Oxford University Press 2002

The moral rights of the author have been asserted

Database right Oxford University Press (maker)

First published 2002

All rights reserved. No part of this publication may be reproduced,
stored in a retrieval system, or transmitted, in any form or by any means,
without the prior permission in writing of Oxford University Press, or as
expressly permitted by law, or under terms agreed with the appropriate
reprographics rights organization. Enquiries concerning reproduction
outside the scope of the above should be sent to the Rights Department,
Oxford University Press, at the address above

You must not circulate this book in any other binding or cover
and you must impose this same condition on any acquirer

A catalogue record for this title is available from the British Library

Library of Congress Cataloging in Publication Data
(Data available)
ISBN 0 19 850858 1

10 9 8 7 6 5 4 3 2 1

Typeset by Cepha Imaging Pvt Ltd
Printed in Great Britain
on acid-free paper by Biddles Ltd, Guildford & King's Lynn

Preface

How many people have not suffered from an episode of pain or itching around their anus? How many of us have not experienced bleeding or noticed a lump after a bowel motion? And has anybody not suffered from a bout of constipation or straining, or even an embarrassing loss of control over his or her bowels?

The fact is that all of us are troubled at some time by our tail ends. For most people this is only an occasional and fleeting problem; and luckily most of these complaints are not serious. But for a large group amongst us, recurring or persistent anal and bowel complaints become a source of irritation, frustration, anxiety, loss of confidence, and even misery.

The causes and treatment of these complaints are often simple and remarkably successful, but fear and embarrassment stop us from seeking out assistance; and ignorance or inexperience on the part of the person whose advice has been sought might result in the entirely wrong advice being given.

Friends and family happily make light of our troubles! Greetings cards trivialize our suffering! But ask anyone who has endured weeks, months, or even years of a painful fissure, protruding haemorrhoids, intractable itching, repeated bleeding, exasperating constipation, or humiliating leakage and all will agree that this is truly no laughing matter.

The aim of this short book is to explain the basis of these all too common complaints and to recommend some simple solutions. No book can ever replace a thorough assessment by a properly trained doctor and warnings about the need to seek medical advice are spread throughout the text. Just the same, many anal and bowel conditions respond well to the simple, common-sense strategies outlined within. I hope you find some relief in the chapters that follow.

Dr Michael Levitt

Contents

1 How the gastrointestinal tract does its job

The fascinating journey from mouth to anus takes anything from a matter of hours to several days depending on many different factors. What we eat and how much, and our levels of physical exercise, stress, and anxiety (and how we each respond to them!), as well as the medications and treatments of various kinds we are prescribed, all influence the workings of our bowels. The presence of certain diseases—gastroenteritis, for example—may also make a big difference.

The beginning

Food is chewed in the mouth to make it possible to swallow, to help savour the taste, and to start the process of digestion by contact with saliva. Once swallowed, food is transmitted rapidly down the gullet (oesophagus) and into the stomach.

Food is temporarily held up by the action of the stomach's muscular outlet channel, the pylorus. This allows food to be exposed to further breakdown by acid and enzymes and it is literally 'churned' into a soft consistency suitable for passage through the remainder of the intestine.

Important steps in the absorption of iron and vitamin B_{12} also occur in the healthy stomach. In the normal state of affairs, stomach content does not go back up into the gullet. When it does—a process called gastro-oesophageal reflux, or often just **reflux**—the acidic stomach content burns the lining of the gullet causing indigestion and other complaints.

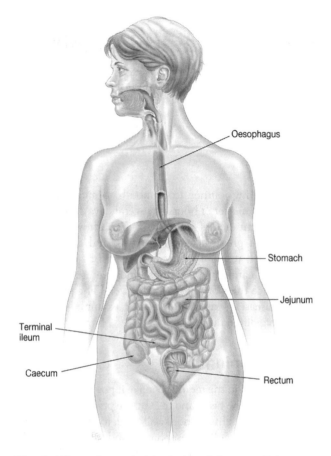

Oesophagus

Stomach

Jejunum

Terminal
ileum

Caecum

Rectum

Fig. 1.1 The entire gastrointestinal tract, from mouth to anus.

The middle

Food remains in the stomach for between one and three
hours. Certain foods, however, tend to slow the stomach's
emptying process and may remain for up to six hours. But
once food leaves the stomach, this quiet life ends. The
small intestine, by contrast, transmits its contents rapidly

by means of vigorous and sustained contraction waves termed 'peristaltic contraction waves' or 'peristalsis'.

The first 30 cm of the small intestine (the duodenum) follow a 270° curve and accept inflow of bile from the liver (to help digest fat) and juices from the pancreas (to help digest carbohydrates and protein). The combined actions of digestive enzymes, acid from the stomach, bile, pancreatic juice, and other secretions mean that intestinal content now bears little resemblance at all to the food eaten often less than one or two hours beforehand.

It is from here on in, however, that the critical work of the gastrointestinal tract—the absorption of nutrients from food—takes place. There are many metres of small intestine (up to ten, depending on how much stretch is put on them!), allowing for a vast, available service for absorption of nutrients. Despite their rapid passage, therefore, plenty of opportunity exists for the required absorption to take place.

The passage of matter through the small intestine ends when its terminal portion (the ileum) pours its contents into the beginning of the large intestine (the caecum). Filling of the caecum starts as early as fifteen minutes after any meal, almost all of which will have been processed and propelled within four hours of eating. The junction between ileum and caecum is called the 'ileo-caecal valve' because it generally does not permit flow of content back into the ileum. Each day, the ileo-caecal valve witnesses the passage of about 1.5 litres of liquid intestinal content literally hurtling into the cavernous caecum.

The end

Unlike the small intestine, the large intestine is an altogether sluggish muscular tube. Propulsion occurs by means of strong, yet rather languid, contraction waves occurring up to six times daily.

These contraction waves—also called 'mass movements'—are generally triggered by the entry of content from the small intestine. They also occur in a regular cycle determined by the interplay of our patterns of eating, sleeping, and exercise. The simple act of getting out of bed in the morning is one of the most predictable triggers for a mass movement. This explains why so many people have to open their bowels first thing in the morning. This cycle of contractions can easily be disturbed if any of these factors is suddenly changed—for example overseas travel or a change in diet.

With each of these mass movements, content of the large intestine is moved further around towards the outlet at the rectum and anus. Obviously, not all of these contractions result in the urge to have a bowel action and it is distension of the left side of the large intestine, especially the sigmoid colon, that accounts for our first urge to open our bowels. Since the large intestine reabsorbs water from its contents, by the time things have reached the rectum—where they can safely be termed **faeces**—they have been well and truly dried out.

In fact, the large intestine is really nothing more than a 'social organ', turning 1.5 litres of unmanageable, wet mush into about 250 g of formed, solid, or at least semi-solid, material—also termed **stool**—that needs to be passed, on average, only once a day.

But if the large intestine is a social organ, then the rectum can be considered a veritable socialite and the anal sphincters the coordinator of proceedings! Our ability to hold on when an urge to open our bowels arrives at an awkward moment is partly because of the special ability of the rectum—the last 15 cm of the large intestine—to relax at first rather than contract on its content. This is supported by active contraction of the anal sphincters, which literally block the escape of rectal contents.

In normal circumstances, we can sense the presence of faeces within the rectum and begin to plan our next evacuation! But, if need be, we can defer, even for a matter of hours. This particular phase is often accompanied by the selective passage of gas—properly termed **flatus**—to reduce the build up of pressure within the rectum and suppress rectal contraction waves. Eventually the force of the large intestine and rectal contraction waves will overwhelm the ability of the anal sphincter muscles to 'hold on' and the need to evacuate becomes urgent.

Evacuation itself is a complex and still incompletely understood process. As we bear down to evacuate, the anal sphincter and pelvic floor muscles relax, opening up the anal canal and permitting passage of faeces under the influence of large intestinal contractions. These may be reinforced by conscious straining of the abdominal muscles. Ideally, evacuation is easy to initiate, easy to complete, and takes only a matter of minutes, leaving the individual comfortably 'empty'. The journey from mouth to anus and beyond is over.

2 The seven elements of a highly effective bowel habit

Most people believe that it is the number of bowel actions per day or per week that determines whether or not their bowel habit is normal. This is simply not so. Although a large majority of individuals do have their bowels open from between three times daily to every third day, there are, amongst these, many who are dissatisfied with their lot. What is more, many perfectly 'normal' people have their bowels open less frequently than every third day.

As it is, nearly all of us experience daily, though subtle, fluctuations of varying degrees in our bowel habit. None of us produce an identical stool two days in a row! There is also a marked difference between men and women: on average, men have their bowels open more often, produce softer faeces, and much more gas than do women, even when eating a similar diet. A large majority of (heterosexual) couples will have made this observation already!

Clearly, how often we have our bowels open varies from person to person and from day to day. What, then, is the correct or ideal bowel habit? The ideal bowel habit should comprise these seven key elements:

(1) the ability to defer a bowel action for a socially acceptable period of time (let's say at least one hour) after the initial urge is experienced, without suffering abdominal or rectal pain as a result;

(2) complete voluntary control over flatus and normally formed faeces;

(3) prompt initiation of evacuation once we sit on the toilet;

(4) smooth, steady passage of faeces over one to two minutes (or less) without pain, bleeding, or protrusion (prolapse);

(5) a sensation of complete rectal emptying upon leaving the toilet;

(6) no rectal or perianal skin symptoms between bowel actions;

(7) no abdominal pain or bloating between bowel actions.

These seven key elements should be achieved without the need for medicines either to speed up or to slow down our intestines. Importantly, these elements make no mention of *how frequently* we should have our bowels open. Clearly, however, these conditions are most likely to be satisfied when we have our bowels open every day or every second day.

What this book is about

Almost all of the common and simple problems people experience with their bowels and bottom ends can be attributed to some interference with these seven key elements. In very many cases the solution is also simple, does not require surgery, and is within easy reach of the sufferers themselves to diagnose and correct.

Many of the difficulties people experience are of their own making, having fallen into bad habits from which they cannot easily return. That is, unless they have an understanding of what it is they are doing wrong! The remedies are generally straightforward and several seemingly different complaints respond to similar strategies.

As you read this book you may prefer to jump ahead to the chapter covering your specific problem—I can certainly appreciate your decision if you are in pain right now! Overall, however, you will probably get a clearer understanding by following the chapters in the order in which they are presented.

Either way, good luck and, most importantly, don't allow any anal and rectal symptoms that do not subside, especially bleeding, to go unseen by a doctor.

3 Urgency and incontinence of faeces

Inability to control one's bowels is amongst the most humiliating experiences an adult is ever likely to encounter. Whilst this is a rare event for most of us—usually only experienced in the course of a bout of food poisoning or gastroenteritis—it may be a recurring nightmare for some.

There are many different causes of anal incontinence, reflecting the interplay of stool frequency and consistency, anal sphincter muscle strength, and the efficiency of rectal emptying. Most sufferers—and very often their doctors—focus on the anal sphincter as the likely culprit: 'My muscles are too weak'; 'I can't seem to shut off my back passage'. Although these highly specialized muscles may be weakened or torn by childbirth, surgery, or trauma, they are often *not* to blame.

Put simply, the anal sphincter mechanism comprises two cylinders of muscle which surround the anal canal, one inside the other and both about 3 cm long. Both muscular cylinders—the internal and external anal sphincters—are continuously active, even when we are asleep. The **internal sphincter** responds only to reflex signals and cannot be made to increase or decrease its 'grip' by conscious effort. It accounts for most of the pressure inside the anus at rest and is, therefore, vital in helping us to maintain minute-to-minute control over flatus.

The **external sphincter**, on the other hand, can be called on to 'squeeze' the anus shut. When we cough,

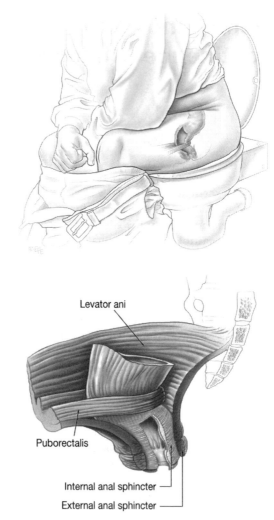

Fig. 3.1 The anal sphincter mechanism.

sneeze, laugh, or experience a strong urge to open our bowels, the external sphincter contracts as a reflex to prevent incontinence. On the other hand, the external sphincter should relax completely when we bear down to evacuate, so permitting the anal canal to open widely. Failure of the external sphincter to *relax* during defaecation may result in the need to strain excessively; failure of the external sphincter to *contract* with sufficient strength, once a need to evacuate arrives, may cause urgency and major incontinence.

Yet failure of the anal sphincter is rarely the main cause of any individual's incontinence. Much more commonly, incontinence of faeces falls into these two main patterns.

Urgency, loose stools, and irritable bowel syndrome

In any individual, the degree of urgency that we experience in association with any one bowel action is a balance between the strength of the anal sphincter muscle and the force with which the bowel motion is delivered into the lower rectum. Even the person with the world's strongest anal sphincters would be unable to resist a column of tap water pumped into the bowel under high pressure! Many of us know from experience that even normal anal sphincters may be overwhelmed by the force of diarrhoea during a bout of gastroenteritis; weakened sphincters may be compromised by nothing more than the effects of a large, spicy meal and a few beers!

In other words, this pattern of urgency and incontinence is much more a reflection of the speed and consistency of our bowel actions than it is of any weakness of our anal sphincter muscles. Typically, such individuals experience great anxiety about going out of the house or into any territory where the location of the nearest toilet is not known to them. In the majority of cases, this is a problem in the morning—one or more bowel actions occurring in succession and becoming progressively looser and more urgent. Afternoons and evenings are generally less 'active' but the pattern is highly variable and may, rarely, even cause overwhelming incontinence during sleep.

Many women comment that their problems often occur while they are out shopping. It seems that the more concerned the individual is about the prospect of an urgent call to the toilet, the more likely such a problem is to happen.

This pattern of urgency and loose stools occurring in an individual in otherwise good health is a typical manifestation of so-called **irritable bowel syndrome**. In such individuals there is overactivity of intestinal propulsion, particularly affecting the large intestine. All the factors that normally provoke large intestinal contractions— getting up in the morning, eating, exercise, anxiety, and stress—seem to provoke *excessive* contractions in these individuals.

Not infrequently the situation is aggravated, if not caused, by dietary factors. Many individuals are thought to have sensitivities to food substances such as dairy products (lactose intolerance) or wheat protein (gluten sensitivity). These diagnoses are frequently made but are rarely proven. What is more, a significant number of those individuals who, at first, improve on special diets designed to eliminate these substances subsequently deteriorate despite rigid adherence to the plan.

In fact, the dietary factors that most commonly aggravate irritable bowel syndrome and provoke urgency and looseness are those we already know to be the cause— alcohol, bran, caffeine, fruit, spices, and vegetables! The dietary and drug treatment of urgency incontinence is detailed in Chapter 12.

Although there may also be some weakness of the anal sphincter mechanism present in these individuals, treatment nearly always requires nothing more than the pursuit of a genuinely solid stool consistency. Using the simple means outlined in Chapter 12, almost all patients with this embarrassing and often distressing complaint can regain control over their bowels and greatly restore social confidence. Of all the patients I have treated with bowel disorders, few are more grateful than those whose incontinence, often extending back decades, is cured by advice that did nothing more than achieve a solid bowel action!

Passive soiling of soft stool

I am frequently consulted by people whose main complaint is the unconscious seepage of soft, paste-like stool. It is usually noted shortly after a bowel action has been completed and is often more noticeable if exercise is undertaken shortly after a bowel action. This soiling soon leads to irritation of the perianal skin causing itching, burning pain, and spotting of blood.

Although this pattern of incontinence occurs in both men and women, it is characteristic of faecal incontinence in men. The pattern is the direct result of a stool consistency that is too soft and which cannot, therefore, be completely expelled. It is *not* primarily the result of a weakened anal sphincter mechanism, especially in men, whose anal sphincters are, in fact, longer and stronger than most women's. Yet men are more likely to suffer from this pattern of faecal incontinence because of their generally faster and softer bowel habits.

Such individuals, whether men or women, frequently recount not only the soft stool consistency, but also the prolonged period of time required to 'wipe up' after a bowel action. Although more than 90 per cent of a bowel action has been passed in a matter of seconds, the residue of soft faeces within the rectum causes a sensation of pelvic pressure and incomplete rectal emptying. Many sheets of toilet paper and many minutes of time are expended in attempts to leave the anus clean and dry. Despite these efforts, a small residue of stool inevitably remains behind.

The presence of even a small amount of faeces within the lower rectum initiates a normal human reflex called 'recto-anal inhibition'. Any stimulation of the lower rectum causes a spontaneous and reflex relaxation of the internal sphincter muscle. This, you will recall, is the sphincter muscle predominantly in charge of unconscious anal control. As these individuals leave the toilet with their residue of soft, sticky faeces, the anus reflexly relaxes, encouraging passive leakage! If these same individuals then set out on some exercise—even a simple walk—the increased intra-abdominal pressure associated with exertion provides above average force which literally 'squeezes' the soft faeces out of their relaxed, open anus.

The solution to this problem rests not with attempts to bolster the anal sphincter mechanism but with the individual being able to achieve more complete rectal emptying. Once again, this can best be achieved by the pursuit of a more solid stool consistency. I have absolutely no doubt that the human gastrointestinal system was designed to operate best where stool resembles the shape and consistency (although not the colour!) of an unripe banana. Soft stool of the consistency of porridge or peanut paste can rarely be expelled completely by the normal, human anorectum. Once evacuation of a solid stool has been initiated, gravity and momentum assist the gentle, undulating rectal contraction waves to expel the stool completely, and leave the rectum empty and the anus instantly clean and dry.

If the rectum is left empty on completion of evacuation there is no risk of passive incontinence occurring; if passive soiling of soft faeces continues to occur, it almost always means that the stool consistency is not yet hard enough. The sure sign that you have got it right is when evacuation of stool is prompt and complete, and the perianal region is immediately 'clean'. This treatment is simple and generally very effective (see Chapter 12 for details of diet and medication).

Occasionally it may be necessary to insert a simple glycerine suppository to assist in cleaning up the last little bit. This is a safe long-term strategy if it proves necessary and is much healthier for you than repeated and prolonged straining or having to insert your own finger to clean out the lower rectum, as do some individuals occasionally feel the need.

The third cause of incontinence— anal sphincter failure

As indicated above, incontinence due to true anal sphincter failure is quite rare. Just the same, the anal sphincter muscles may be torn by difficult childbirth (see Chapter 10), divided in the process of anal surgery or penetrating trauma, or damaged by severe infection. The sphincter mechanism may also be stretched by repeated rectal protrusion (rectal prolapse—see Chapter 5) or weakened by nerve damage sustained during prolonged or difficult vaginal delivery (see Chapter 10).

This pattern of incontinence is characterized by more total incontinence, even to formed or solid stool. There may be urgency incontinence (inability to make it to the toilet in time), passive incontinence (unconscious leakage between bowel actions), and incontinence to flatus. If there is true rectal prolapse, the individual may also be aware of the protrusion of a large amount of rectal tissue during defaecation, at other times, or even continuously.

In this group of patients, specialist evaluation is important in case a surgically correctable problem does exist. The conditions most likely to respond to surgery are a complete sphincter tear due to obstetric trauma and complete rectal prolapse. Even in cases where the sphincter is genuinely at fault, the basic rules for the treatment of incontinence apply: *keep the stool solid and the rectum empty*.

Summary: A simple guide to treating urgency and incontinence

1. Achieve a consistently solid stool (see Chapter 12):

    (a) Reduce dietary intake of softening and stimulating foods.

    (b) Consider regular and/or occasional anti-diarrhoeal medication.

2. If experiencing difficulty evacuating solid stool, assist rectal emptying with glycerine suppositories.

3. Persistent incontinence of genuinely solid stool requires assessment by your family doctor.

4. Surgery may be of benefit when:

    (a) There has been a tear in the sphincter muscle mechanism due to childbirth.

    (b) There is full thickness rectal prolapse.

    (c) The anal sphincter has been severely damaged by infection or repeated surgery.

4
Constipation and straining

Occasional constipation is almost universal. Even recurring or continuing constipation is common, and, predictably, women are more likely to be affected, having, on average, a naturally more sluggish bowel than do men. Whenever there is an unexpected change in bowel habit (especially in the over-50 age group), careful consideration must be given to excluding serious causes such as colonic cancer. Your doctor is undoubtedly the best person to advise on these matters; this is not something that should be deferred or for which alternative therapies should be tried before you have excluded potentially dangerous causes.

The word 'constipation' means different things to different people. For some it is a matter of feeling infrequent urges to have their bowels open and the need to take ever increasing doses of opening medicines to get their bowels working. For others it is primarily a problem of difficulty with emptying their rectum, making them strain vigorously on the toilet, even when their stool is soft.

For others, constipation is an infuriating combination of both infrequent bowel actions and the need to strain excessively.

Few physical complaints are as misunderstood by both the majority of people and health workers alike as is constipation. Few conditions are as shrouded in myth or have as much guilt for its existence attributed to the sufferer. But there *is* a way forward and it is fairly simple. It starts with establishing the nature of your problem: the type of constipation that you have.

Slow transit constipation ('sluggish colon')

A generally slow and sluggish colon may be due to a number of quite correctable diseases or due to the use of numerous medications. When constipation appears after many years of a more normal bowel habit, these possibilities must always be considered and a thorough assessment by your family doctor is essential.

At the end of the day, however, most constipation due to a sluggish colon is a transient problem only and can be attributed to something simple like a recent change in diet, a change in life situation (new job, less exercise), or even the effect of long-distance travel. As a rule, we are familiar with these effects and know that attention to fluid and fibre in our diet or a single dose of a strong laxative will generally correct the problem.

For some of us—mainly women—care has to be taken on a daily basis to keep fibre and fluid intake at high levels. If not, constipation due to slow transit and hard stools becomes a significant problem. I am sure many of you fit into this category.

For others, the degree of constipation is worse still and fibre alone isn't always enough. From time to time, such individuals need to take stronger laxatives if they are to avoid—and sometimes overcome—a major hold-up. As a result, there may be wild fluctuations, from constipation, building up over days or weeks, to diarrhoea in the wake of an occasional dose of laxative.

Rather than continue this pattern of ups and downs, you might consider one of the 'intermediate' group of laxatives; these are the sweet syrups lactulose and sorbitol, which are particularly useful as they are *not* habit forming. They do, however, result in considerable gas production, which many people find annoying and even uncomfortable.

Nevertheless, they are clearly safer than many of the other available laxatives—particularly the herbal laxatives, which tend to result in complete dependence upon them for any sort of bowel action at all. Herbal laxatives contain such substances as senna, cascara, and frangula bark. Your local pharmacist will be able to advise you on which laxatives are of this herbal, habit-forming variety.

Then there are those individuals whose constipation has progressed into the 'professional ranks'. For those of you with an even slower, more sluggish, colon, fibre simply isn't enough. In fact, in this group, dietary fibre often only aggravates bloating and abdominal discomfort.

Genuine slow transit constipation occurs almost entirely in women (95 per cent of cases). It may date from adolescence or even early childhood. Sometimes it develops after seemingly unrelated abdominal or pelvic surgery or is provoked by severe illness or injury. Infrequent urges to defaecate, laxative dependence, and painful abdominal bloating are the predominant complaints.

Well-intentioned doctors, pharmacists, physiotherapists, and family friends will all insist that 'you're not eating enough fibre!' Filled with guilt and pessimism you return to the natural bran, psyllium husks, multigrain breads, bowls of salad, and piles of vegetables you have already been swallowing for months and even years without effect. But what do you get? Painful bloating by flatus that will not pass! More fibre than a horse eats and still, they say, you can't be having enough.

Or water! That's it, you're not drinking enough water. So off you go and drink your three litres of distilled water a day, until, drowning in water and unable to keep your bladder empty for more than an hour, someone tells you, 'try these, they're great and they're natural!'

Ah ha! The herbal laxative! Your new weapon in the fight against constipation and, yes, what a difference it makes. OK, there's a bit of abdominal cramping and the stool does tend to catch you on the hop, but wow! You can go so much more easily, and every day too.

At least, you can for a while. Soon the laxative doesn't seem to be quite as effective or quite so predictable. You increase the dose, three tablets instead of two, another centimetre of the chewy bar. Perhaps you should try a different one? Or maybe the two in combination? What about taking them morning *and* night? And there's still that one in the medicine cabinet that Grandma used to take.

Soon the colon is hooked, totally addicted to these herbal laxatives. But they don't always work reliably and when they eventually do—after a doubling of dose or yet another change in the laxative 'cocktail'—the force with which the bowel action appears causes painful abdominal cramps which may be so great as to cause embarrassing leakage or, worse, substantial incontinence.

By the time many constipated patients get to my surgery, they have spent many months and often years completely bedevilled by their bowels. When will their bowels next open? Will this laxative work today? Should they try another one? Can they leave home now or should they wait at home until the laxatives do work?

Their lives revolve around if and when and how a bowel action might be achieved. They are truly disabled, convinced that they are somehow at fault, embarrassed to discuss their complaints and, quite often, thoroughly miserable. The term 'lazy bowel' says it all: it's *your* fault; *you* are doing it all wrong!

How do you escape from this vicious cycle?

The first step in getting things right is to get a few facts straight! There are many myths about how our bowels should work which get in the way of helping constipated people overcome or live with their problem.

Myth no. 1: 'I don't want laxatives; my bowels should work naturally'

So many people that I see are convinced that their bowels should—no, must—work without outside help. Ingrained in their minds from an early age and reinforced by the modern push to eat more fibre, they struggle to accept the need to use 'medication' to get their bowels working. I often hear the words 'I want to be normal'; even more frequently, women tell me, 'I want to be able to go like him', referring, of course, to their partner.

Yet shouldn't all of our bodily systems work without the need for outside help? Ask yourself: Do people with high blood pressure, angina, arthritis, or asthma also reject all medication? Rarely, if ever! The difference is that many people simply don't regard constipation, or other bowel-related problems, as valid or real. Like so many of the conditions covered in this book, they are a bit of a joke and not to be taken seriously. Meanwhile, the sufferer is left feeling ashamed and alone.

So the first step in getting the better of your constipation is to accept that this *is* a valid condition, that it is *not* your fault, and that some form of treatment *is* required. If you are in any doubt as to how significant and how real your constipation is, ask yourself this simple question: 'Have my problems with getting my bowels to work begun to affect my enjoyment of life?' If the answer is 'yes', then some form of medication is surely worth considering.

Myth no. 2: 'If it's herbal, it's natural and that's OK'

By the time people seek out a specialist, they have generally been experimenting with laxatives for a long while and there is no doubt that the easiest and quickest results come from herbal preparations and other stimulant laxatives (for example bisacodyl). These cause the muscle in the bowel wall to contract and to propel its contents towards the rectum. They act on the bowel wall whether or not there are faeces within. Such contractions often cause cramping abdominal pain.

But the downside to these laxatives is that the bowel wall muscle becomes progressively less able to respond to all the stimuli that normally make it contract, such as getting up in the morning, physical exercise, and eating.

Even worse, the bowel needs progressively more of these laxatives to get the desired result. Herbal and other stimulant laxatives are not, in themselves, poisonous and they are not considered pre-cancerous; they simply and steadily render your colon ever more flaccid and unresponsive, and this may be irreversible.

Herbal and other stimulant laxatives are useful 'one-off' agents for occasional constipation. They may, in some poeple, be the *only* agents that work, but, as a general rule, they should be avoided in the long-term management of constipation.

Myth no. 3: 'I must open my bowels every day'

This is another 'untruth' passed down from generation to generation and deeply ingrained in Western society. For most men, it is achieved without a second thought and perhaps it is men, believing that theirs is the 'right' way, who have promulgated this myth in the past. Nowadays the fibre lobby has joined the brigade insisting on a 'daily, soft, formed, floating stool'. Really!

As I indicated in Chapter 2, the ideal bowel habit is not defined by how frequently we go but by how easily and how completely. Similarly, constipation is not best defined by how infrequently we go but by how much distress these infrequent bowel actions cause us. I have seen many patients whose bowels work only every four days (even up to one week) and who satisfy all the seven elements of a highly effective bowel habit. In short, these individuals are not constipated; they are normal!

The most damaging aspect of this myth is that it drives constipated people to take laxatives on a daily basis. This is a sure recipe for rapidly inducing laxative dependence, a progressively less responsive colon, and a steady rise in laxative use.

But many people may have insufficient food and bowel matter in the system even to generate a satisfactory daily stool. This is often the case in young, figure-conscious women or older people whose appetites have diminished with age.

Hence, the bowel action effected by the daily laxative seems small and unsatisfactory. Perspective is lost and laxative use increases in search of a more substantial result!

Many people do *not* have their bowels open daily.

Many more people who do not have their bowels open daily do not *need* to do so and can safely give up the pointless struggle to satisfy a 'rule' that really should not apply.

Almost all seriously constipated people who take regular laxatives need only take them every two to three days or, preferably, even less frequently.

Of all the myths that apply to the treatment of constipation, the belief that we should have our bowels open every day is the hardest to overcome and is the basis of the single, most important step in treatment.

A four-step treatment plan for slow transit constipation

Step 1: Do I have a sluggish colon?

Having read the description of slow transit constipation, you have to ask yourself: 'Is this my problem?' The characteristic scenario is:

(1) long-standing constipation;

(2) infrequent urges to defaecate;

(3) dependence on laxative medications;

(4) painful abdominal bloating.

Other features worth re-emphasizing are the strong female preponderance and the tendency for fibre to aggravate abdominal pain and bloating. If you are not sure—and especially if your constipation is a recent development—you must check with your family doctor. Your doctor can help exclude more sinister causes and, if appropriate, arrange investigations to determine which type of constipation you do have.

Step 2: Avoid excessive fibre

By the time your constipation has reached the First Division (let alone the Premier League), your colon will not respond to a mild laxative such as a fibre supplement. The large intestine will laugh at these puny efforts to make it contract while all the time permitting gas to build up inside.

So yes, it is OK! You have permission: you do *not* need to take more fibre. In fact, if you are brave, you should even take less.

Step 3: Take your laxatives less often

This is the big hurdle and it is mainly a psychological barrier that you need to overcome. *Do not take laxatives daily.* Set yourself a simple goal and take them only every second day, but be disciplined. If you are serious about restoring some sense of control over your bowels you will persevere.

Once you have broken the cycle of daily laxative use you are well and truly on the way to mastering your sluggish colon. Having settled on second daily laxatives and survived (against all predictions!), push the limits a bit further still and try taking them every third day. You will respond, it will be a more substantial result, and you've got two days all to yourself before you have to worry about your bowels again!

Gradually, you may have the confidence to stretch the gap between doses even further. But you have already won the most important battle; and, in any event, you will probably need to implement Step 4 before going much further.

Step 4: Move towards osmotic laxatives

Even when taken only every third or fourth day, herbal and other stimulant laxatives create a dependent colon and abdominal cramping. The next challenge is gradually to move away from these laxatives to those of the osmotic variety. These are sweet syrups—lactulose and sorbitol—and concentrated salts such as Epsom salts (magnesium sulphate).

For the seriously constipated individual already dependent upon herbal and other stimulant laxatives, the milder sweet syrups are unlikely to be effective; only the more powerful salts will work. All of the salts are unpalatable and most people have to disguise them with cordial or juice to get them down. Overall, I have found that patients regard Epsom salts as the easiest to use although others, such as Golytely, Fleet oral, Colon Cleanse, and Picolax, can be used.

Rather than make a direct switch from herbal to osmotic, I recommend a more gradual transition. Continue with your third daily dose of herbal or stimulant laxative but add one level teaspoonful of Epsom salts dissolved in a large glass of water with cordial added 'to taste'. As you gain confidence in this new regime, reduce the amount of herbal laxative and substitute with more Epsom salts. Gradually you will be able to wean yourself off all herbal laxatives and manage only with Epson salts.

You might ask, 'What is the point if I still need to take an opening medicine?' The fact is that is doesn't really matter if you stay on herbal laxatives forever—they are not dangerous! But the advantage of a switch to osmotic laxatives is the prospect of stretching out the time between doses to one week, and the real possibility of the return of some spontaneous bowel activity.

When patients of mine have been able to follow these steps and are taking salts on a once- or twice-a-week basis, they frequently report the return of some spontaneous bowel activity between doses. No, they almost never get back to 'normal'. But the colon is capable of some recovery even after years of laxative abuse, and a gradual reduction in the dose of Epsom salts may yet be possible.

Either way, you are back in control of your bowels and not the reverse!

Summary: A four-step treatment plan for severe slow transit constipation

1. Do I have a sluggish colon?
2. Avoid excessive fibre.
3. Take laxatives less often.
4. Move towards osmotic laxatives.

Disorders of rectal evacuation

Satisfactory rectal evacuation is a complex process. It depends upon the timely concurrence of a forceful colonic contraction, a well-formed stool, and appropriate relaxation of the pelvic floor and sphincter muscles. Difficulty in achieving satisfactory emptying of the rectum can be the result of a wide range of underlying problems. Common to all of them is the excessive straining to get things out. For those of you in the grip of a major disorder of rectal evacuation, a visit to the toilet can be an exhausting and exasperating ordeal.

Disorders of evacuation can be conveniently separated into:

(1) disorders of initiation ('can't get things started'); and

(2) disorders of completion ('can't finish the job').

You will probably immediately recognize into which group you fit; fortunately they don't usually overlap.

Disorders of initiation

There are numerous causes for such a problem. Some are simple to understand and fairly easy to recognize, both by you, the sufferer, and by your doctor. A painful anal condition (see Chapter 5) or a fixed narrowing of the anal canal, usually following prior anal or rectal surgery, are straightforward to diagnose and to treat.

Likewise, if you have a degree of slow transit constipation you may be presenting your rectum with a slow-moving, dehydrated bowel motion, a veritable rock that no normal anus can successfully expel!

But most causes of this complaint—and certainly the most intriguing—are largely behavioural! In other words, they stem from faulty patterns of both toileting (going at the wrong time) and defaecation (failing to relax the pelvic floor when straining at stool).

The act of defaecation is a very private one. Few of us are comfortable about sharing the noises and odours of a bowel action with even our closest family members, let alone with the public at large. This makes us wary of when and where we permit ourselves to go. As a result, we may be inclined to sit on the toilet well in advance of the natural urge so we can 'empty' our bowels at a time when we can guarantee privacy. For example, many people will instigate a bowel action in the morning—usually involving a lengthy sit on the toilet with reading material—rather than risk having to go later on in the day while at work either in the office or out and about 'in the field'.

I call this 'pre-empting' a bowel action. Is it any wonder at all, then, that such a bowel action will be prolonged and will require excessive straining when it takes place in the complete absence of the normal intestinal contractions vital for satisfactory evacuation!

We can now add yet another myth about how our bowels should work.

Myth no. 4: 'Never delay the urge to open your bowels'

Many people are brought up to believe that failure to respond promptly to an urge to defaecate will inevitably result in constipation. Wrong! The human rectum—and I hope you will pardon my bias—is a particularly clever part of the intestines. Unlike the remainder of the gastrointestinal tract, small and large, the rectum has the ability to 'relax receptively'. In other words, it can fill with contents without attempting to expel them by contracting. This is an essential function if we are to fulfil Step 1 of the seven elements outlined in Chapter 2, namely the ability to defer a bowel action for a socially appropriate length of time. In short, the rectum—in combination with the anal sphincters—is a highly social organ designed specifically to allow us to put off that first urge if it occurs at an inconvenient time or if it isn't a particularly strong urge.

Sitting in the bathroom in response to an indifferent urge to defaecate—I call this 'speculating'—is another sure recipe for difficulty in initiating a bowel action. The longer we can delay that decision to go to the toilet to open our bowels, the greater the pressure that will have built up inside the colon and rectum and the more natural the force will be to help initiate expulsion of faeces.

Conversely, the less forceful the innate urge is for us to go, the more voluntary straining you will need to employ and the more likely your stool is to get stuck in 'no-man's land'! Imagine the confusion inside your rectum when you start straining at a time when it simply isn't ready to respond! Sure, you can, with enough effort, expel some material but the result will never match the effort.

An interesting problem encountered in the process of pre-empting, speculating, and straining is that of paradoxical contraction (rather than relaxation) of the pelvic floor muscles and the external anal sphincters when attempting to evacuate the rectum. Instead of these muscles relaxing—which allows the anus to open up and the angle between anus and rectum to straighten, favouring evacuation of rectal contents—they contract. This narrows and angulates the exit passage, creating a very real sensation of blockage or obstruction. We call this 'obstructed defaecation' or 'puborectalis paradox'.

The more speculative the visit to the toilet and the less natural the force behind the bowel action, the more some voluntary straining is required and the greater is the likelihood of paradoxical contraction and 'obstruction'. Despite the absence of any true mechanical blockage, individuals afflicted with this problem are utterly convinced that there is one. Why else would faeces not come out? And why do they appear flattened, like a ribbon, when they do come out?

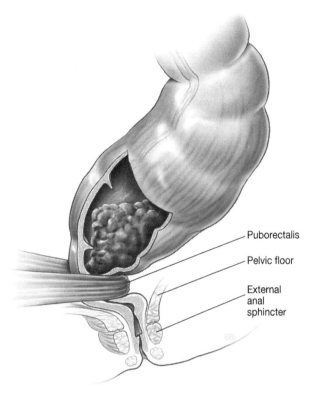

Puborectalis

Pelvic floor

External
anal
sphincter

Fig. 4.1 Paradoxical contraction—rather than relaxation—of the external anal sphincter, pelvic floor and puborectalis muscles during evacuation narrows and angulates the anorectal junction 'obstructing' the anal outlet.

A four-step treatment plan for easing evacuation

Step 1: Exclude the obvious

If you are in pain or if your symptoms have appeared after previous anal surgery such as a haemorrhoidectomy, seek the advice of your family doctor.

Step 2: Ensure adequate colonic speed

If you have even a small degree of slow colonic transit, any associated difficulties with initiating rectal evacuation will be made far worse. In order that you are able to start evacuation with relative ease, it is vital to ensure that colonic contents are moving reasonably quickly.

The advice already provided in this chapter about slow transit constipation is, therefore, also relevant here. For milder degrees of slow transit, a regular fibre supplement or a mild osmotic laxative such as lactulose syrup should suffice. For more extreme cases of slow colonic transit, more powerful agents may be required.

Step 3: The three Ds

If, on the other hand, your problems with initiating evacuation have nothing at all to do with easily correctable anorectal pathology or genuine slow transit constipation, you are probably engaging in excessive voluntary straining and may well be either pre-empting or speculating at least some of the time. The solution to your problem rests with retraining yourself towards a more effective pattern of evacuation. This is summarized as the three Ds.

1. *Defer or delay* defaecation. Learn to hold on rather than respond to the first urge. The more intense the urge is, the easier you will find it to initiate a bowel action. It is much better to hold on and delay a bowel action, for example because you don't want to go in 'public',[1] than it is to sit down and try well in advance of a strong urge.

2. *Desist* from futile straining. Inevitably, you will make a mistake! And especially so early on. Remember that it takes many months and years to develop the sort of behavioural pattern that is causing your problem with

---

[1] *When are the designers of public access buildings going to emerge from the era of the Roman Empire and build conveniences that permit us some privacy?*

evacuation—it will certainly take many weeks or months to undo it!

But when you do go to the toilet and find that nothing will come out, do not sit and strain. So, too bad, you got it wrong this time. Add this experience to your 'database' and know that next time you won't respond until a more appropriate urge occurs. Futile straining is not good for you and you simply have to accept that you chose the wrong time to go. Get up and walk away 'clean'.

3. *Distinguish* between weak (false) and strong (real) urges. It is important to learn from experience which sensations are likely to end up in a successful visit to the toilet and which sensations are merely going to result in futile struggling and straining. In time, it should be possible to recognize a false urge for what it is and ignore it, awaiting the 'real thing'. In short, never go to the toilet to open your bowels unless you are certain that you have urgent and pressing business to do!

Step 4: Suppositories—worth a try

If your rectum is loaded and you cannot effect any evacuation, you may become very uncomfortable indeed. You may have a constant sensation of heaviness and fullness in the rectum, the urge to defaecate, and even outright pain. You may also be experiencing a tendency to leak soft faeces around a great ball of more solid material. This is an ideal situation in which to try suppositories. I suggest that you insert one or two simple glycerine suppositories, which act as a lubricant and softener to help get that ball 'rolling'.

There are other suppositories available—most notably containing bisacodyl (Duralax, Bisalax, Dulcolax), which are more active since they provoke local rectal contraction. Some people find them more effective but they may produce painful rectal spasms that often linger after evacuation has been achieved. And, in the long term, they may also induce tolerance—the need to take more and more just to have the same effect.

Summary: A four-step treatment plan for easing evacuation

1. Exclude the obvious (pain and stricture).
2. Ensure adequate colonic speed (diet or laxatives).
3. The three Ds
   (a) *Defer*—until the urge is strong.
   (b) *Desist*—from futile straining.
   (c) *Distinguish*—between real and false urges.
4. Suppositories—worth a try.

Disorders of completion

Failure to evacuate the rectum completely is an almost universal human experience! As already discussed in Chapter 3, this is almost always the result of having too soft a stool consistency; not surprisingly, it is very common amongst men.

Typically these individuals have no great difficulty initiating a bowel action, since their stool is soft and generally quite fast moving. Most of 'the job' is done within a matter of seconds but the soft faeces literally break off halfway out leaving pasty material precariously attached to the perianal skin and a similar residue literally marooned inside the lower rectum! This creates a clear awareness of rectal fullness or pressure, sometimes described as an urge to bear down. Whatever the description, the unmistakable conclusion is that 'the job' has not been finished.

In this situation, straining might enable some more faecal material to descend and repeated wiping retrieves a small additional amount of this residue. Sufferers frequently describe 'difficulty wiping up' or complain that they 'go through half a roll of paper' at each visit to the toilet. Once again, blame is cast at the anal sphincter muscles: 'My anal muscles won't close'; or at nearby skin tags: 'Those skin tags get in the way'.

In frustration these individuals leave the bathroom sensing that evacuation has not been complete and having wiped their poor rear end raw. As discussed in Chapter 3, the problem here is virtually always one of an excessively soft stool and nothing at all to do with skin tags or major sphincteric weakness. Normal human rectal evacuation depends heavily on the presence of a solid, intact stool—'the big banana'—to enable it to be complete. The colonic and rectal contraction wave is strong enough to initiate evacuation, possibly with the aid of a little voluntary straining, but it is gravity and the momentum of the bit halfway out that drag out the other bit still halfway in!

There can be no doubt that we were intended to pass solid material and not the unformed 'porridge' (or worse) that is characteristic of our high fibre era. The steps necessary to overcome this troublesome problem are very simple and are similar to the advice offered for those with incontinence as well as those with difficulty initiating evacuation. Simple as they are, these steps are highly effective.

A four-step treatment plan for completing rectal evacuation

Step 1: Rule out any serious causes

A sensation of incomplete rectal emptying may be a subtle early sign of rectal inflammation, ulceration, or tumour, especially if there is associated bleeding. A simple examination by your family doctor should exclude these more serious conditions.

Step 2: Keep your stool solid

This can be achieved either by dietary means or with anti-diarrhoeal medication (Chapter 12). You will know you have got it right when evacuation of a formed stool leaves you feeling comfortably empty and the perianal skin clean 'first time'.

Step 3: Defer defaecation until the urge is strong

As your stool firms up you will inevitably need to open your bowels *less* often. If you don't await a forceful urge you may find yourself resorting to bad habits such as speculating when the urge is only mild or pre-empting to avoid a bowel action at a later time. These will result in increasing difficulties initiating a bowel habit.

So for *all* of us at *all* times, hold on until the urge is strong. A *solid stool accompanied by a powerful urge is an ideal recipe for satisfactory rectal evacuation.*

Step 4: Just in case, have some suppositories handy

Whenever recommending that people actively pursue a more solid stool, I need to be mindful of the possibility of them going 'too far'. If getting your stool solid—and there is no doubt that this is the ideal—means that you cannot expel anything at all, don't immediately rush off and take a laxative by mouth. This will certainly get things moving again but will also produce a return to the soft stool consistency that lay at the heart of your original problem.

Rather, insert one or two glycerine suppositories to get the lower bowel empty and reconsider the strategies you have been using to get things solid. Perhaps you can find a better balance and a slightly less solid stool.

Remember, glycerine suppositories are simple lubricants and have no long-term adverse effect. You can use them every day, if necessary, without concern.

Summary: A four-step treatment plan for completing rectal evacuation

1. Rule out any serious causes.

2. Keep your stool solid.

3. Defer defaecation until the urge is strong.

4. Just in case, have some suppositories handy.

Constipation and eating disorders

How often we have our bowels open and how much faeces we actually produce owe a lot to what and how much we eat. I doubt that anyone reading this book hasn't suffered from a slowing of his or her own bowels because of reduced intake of food. Whether this is due to loss of appetite in the course of an illness or as a result of dieting to lose weight, it makes little difference—if you eat less you 'poo' less!

There are, in addition, some disturbing similarities between some forms of constipation and the well-known eating disorders especially anorexia nervosa. There are many theories as to why people—usually young women—quite literally starve themselves in order to lose weight. This may start off as a legitimate weight loss programme or as a means of subconsciously controlling themselves and their environment. Whatever the initial reason, it soon gets out of control; perspective is lost, a distorted body image develops, and a dangerous search for a clearly unattractive bodily appearance ensues.

There are also people suffering from constipation—again, usually young women—whose problematic bowel habit relates to an inadequate diet. Whilst these individuals manage to maintain a satisfactory body weight, they fail to make the obvious connection between what it is that they are *not* eating and why they have such infrequent bowel actions. Since they perceive that they should be producing much more, they strive to do so by taking laxatives instead of correcting their faulty diet.

Herbal laxatives—and others of the stimulant variety—are the easiest to take and they provoke crampy pains and loose stools. But taking a laxative doesn't actually put more matter into the intestines! The end result still fails to satisfy unreasonable expectations of what the bowel is able to produce. With repeated use, these laxatives create ever more difficulty in achieving spontaneous bowel function and a genuine dependence upon laxatives comes to complicate and compound the original issues of inadequate diet and distorted 'stool image'.

I am afraid to say that this particular group of individuals generally remains somewhat disordered in their perception and in their diet for life! Fortunately, constipation itself is not a major threat to life or limb. But I have seen many such people whose unsatisfactory diet and never-ending search for 'the perfect stool' have seen them continue to suffer even after undergoing quite radical surgery. Reassurance, competent advice about laxative options, and repeated encouragement to see the connection between inadequate diet and inadequate bowel habit are all that should be offered.

I have also observed a tendency in some children with constipation—both female and male—to manipulate their parents by virtue of their failure to have their bowels open with sufficient frequency. Undoubtedly there is a degree of true slow colonic transit to start with, but the combination of a vulnerable, somewhat passive child and an intense, over-protective parent or parents results in a downward spiral of repeatedly seeking medical attention, hospitalization, time off school, and, occasionally, major surgery.

This is a difficult situation. The fraught parents demand a solution while the usually healthy-looking child observes the battle between parent and doctor with a surprising lack of concern about his or her own situation. An endless search for the 'right' doctor and the 'magic cure' leads to a damaging cycle of investigation and treatment. Somewhere along the way, a well-intentioned doctor will be manipulated by the powerful combination of a child-in-suffering, irate, even guilt-ridden, parents, and proceed with treatment not really in the best interests of the patient him- or herself.

The solution for all concerned—doctors, parents, and patient—is to await with patience the onset of puberty and adolescence. At this stage, patients will take control of their own destiny, no longer prepared to share the workings of their bowels with anyone, not even their parents. The therapeutic relationship is simplified—patient and doctor only—and the standard option of laxative therapy becomes much more appealing than surgery with all its attendant risks and scars! A whole new range of leisure and social options open up and the sick role no longer holds as much appeal.

This is not to say that these young people do not have a legitimate problem with constipation. They nearly always do and may take it with them for life. It is simply a matter of appreciating the powerful hold that this may give them over their environment, particularly if their parents acquiesce by over-reacting. From the children's perspective, having their parents go into battle for them is highly rewarding, often enough to discourage them from adjusting a little better to their chronic bowel problem. Keep them at school, keep them out of hospital, and avoid surgery wherever possible.

Constipation and childhood abuse

There is increasing recognition of the association between various forms of constipation—both slow transit and disordered evacuation—and traumatic childhood or adolescent experiences. As many as 50 per cent of severely constipated women describe significant abuse—sexual, physical, or emotional—occurring in early life.

How these traumatic experiences affect gastrointestinal function is not clear. Some therapists in this area believe it represents an attempt on the part of the victims literally to 'hold on' to their emotions (as well as their bowels), as if letting go would release memories with which they could not cope. For some constipated individuals these unpleasant past events have been kept hidden for many years, even from their spouses and children. On numerous occasions I have found that gentle enquiry about childhood experiences has been rewarded with the first 'public' admission of long-suppressed unhappiness.

This is not to say that all, or even the majority of, constipated individuals have suffered abuse in their youth. Nor does the painful process of reliving and, hopefully, reconciling past abuse correct the associated constipation. But the suppressed anger and fear, the guilt and low self-esteem that accompany constipation after such trauma often create many other problems. Difficulty maintaining relationships, chronic anxiety states, and depression are common. For these problems to improve, if not the constipation, recognition of the long past initiating events and expert counselling are essential.

As you read this, you may for the first time make the connection between your own bowel problems and abuse suffered as a child or adolescent. Your family doctor will be aware of this association and will be able to advise you about the best available counselling services. If you are embarrassed or uncomfortable about approaching your usual family doctor—perhaps because they may know or have treated the offending and abusive person— find another doctor, possibly in another part of town.

Getting to understand the source of your symptoms is absolutely vital if the process of healing and recovery from abuse is to start. So make that first move—for yourself— as soon as you can.

5
Pain, bleeding, piles, and prolapse

Anal pain. Rectal bleeding. Perianal prolapse and swelling. These are amongst the most common human physical complaints. And why not? Almost everyone on earth has an anus and each of us uses it, often on numerous occasions every day. Luckily for doctors working in this field, the range of possible causes for these complaints is small making diagnosis relatively easy. Even luckier, for the sufferers of anal pain, bleeding, piles, and prolapse, their causes are rarely serious.

Yet the vast majority of people prefer to suffer in silence rather than disclose this most private part of their anatomy. Home remedies, expensive over-the-counter creams or suppositories and horror stories about surgical treatment abound. Doctors themselves have little training in the diagnosis and treatment of these conditions, and misdiagnosis, though rarely serious, is common. Almost all of these anal complaints tend, at some stage to be labelled 'haemorrhoids', resulting in unnecessary prolongation of symptoms and undue expense.

The truth is that haemorrhoids do, from time to time, cause all of these symptoms. But the clinical features of most common anal conditions are surprisingly consistent. On the basis of the descriptions that follow, you should be able to diagnose your own problem.

But first, an important warning! Rectal bleeding of any degree, whether fresh blood or old, must be assessed by your doctor before assuming that the cause is not a serious one. Bleeding is a characteristic symptom of rectal tumours, both benign polyps and cancers, which can be readily excluded on the basis of a careful interview and a gentle internal examination. Your doctor can then determine whether or not more detailed testing is necessary.

Although the vast majority of people with rectal bleeding do have nothing more than minor anal disease, it is essential that this symptom (above all others) is assessed by your doctor.

Haemorrhoids

The term haemorrhoids—also called 'piles'—is one with which we are all familiar and many people even use these words in general conversation. But apart from knowing that it refers, in general, to the anus, very few people know what a haemorrhoid really is. Even many doctors diagnose anal complaints as 'haemorrhoids' when none are present or, if present, are not the cause of the symptoms.

So what are haemorrhoids?

At the upper end of the anal canal—where anus and rectum meet—the moist, smooth lining of the bowel bulges, usually at three points, to form what are called the anal 'cushions'. These cushions are the result of an expansion of the tissue immediately beneath the surface lining made up of a mixture of elastic tissue and small blood vessels. These cushions lie in contact with each other sealing off the upper anus and helping us to keep control over gas. In short, anal cushions are normal structures that form part of the normal closure mechanism of the anus.

Under the influence of a variety of factors—constipation and straining, menstruation, and pregnancy—these cushions can become congested and enlarged. It is these enlarged anal cushions that are correctly called haemorrhoids.

Haemorrhoids commonly bleed or protrude (prolapse) or both, usually during and immediately after a bowel action.

(a)

(b)

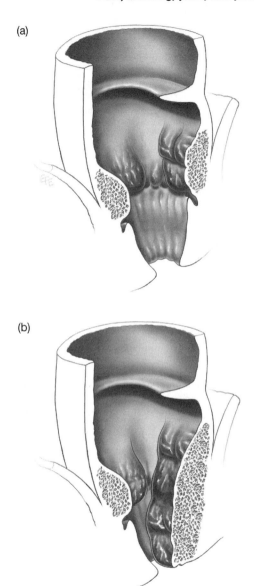

Fig. 5.1 Haemorrhoids arise at the upper end of the anal canal but can slide down and protrude when they become large.

(c)

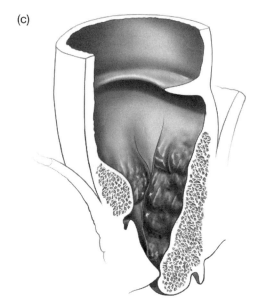

Fig. 5.1 *(Continued)*

The passage of stool compresses and traumatizes the haemorrhoids provoking the bleeding. This bleeding is bright red—obviously 'fresh'. The blood may be noticed on the toilet paper or may be seen dripping into the toilet bowl after the stool has passed. There may even be spraying of this bright red blood around the bowl.

Haemorrhoidal bleeding is not dark—as would occur from a vein—and haemorrhoids are most definitely not a type of varicose vein. This myth has long been disproven but remains folk law in society at large and, sadly, is still so described in some current medical textbooks. Many people still believe that people with varicose veins in their legs are more prone to suffer from haemorrhoids. This is also quite untrue!

When haemorrhoids become even larger, they can literally slide down the anal canal and protrude externally.

This is called prolapse. Prolapse usually occurs in the process of having a bowel action but can occur when the individual is squatting or during exertion such as lifting heavy objects. A prolapsing haemorrhoid generally retreats to its proper, internal location of its own accord. When particularly large, however, they may need gentle manual assistance to do so. Only when very large indeed do haemorrhoids become permanently prolapsed. In this situation they may bleed on contact with underwear, discharge mucus, and cause both itching and general discomfort.

Repeated prolapse over weeks and months can lead to the formation of an external, perianal skin tag. This is an untidy, irregular flap of skin around the anal opening which does not go back inside even when the haemorrhoid itself does. Many people are aware of these skin tags, which can be readily felt when wiping up after a bowel action. Skin tags are often mistakenly called haemorrhoids. They are not haemorrhoids; in this case they are just the perianal skin's reaction to repeated prolapse of a haemorrhoid.

From time to time haemorrhoids may undergo acute thrombosis (clotting) resulting in sudden pain associated with protrusion. Haemorrhoids, however, rarely explain long-standing anal pain or anal pain of a frequently recurring nature. In short, where anal pain is the predominant symptom, haemorrhoids are unlikely to be the explanation. Equally, painless bright red rectal bleeding that occurs with a bowel action strongly suggests a diagnosis of haemorrhoids.

What causes haemorrhoids?

Given that all of us have anal cushions, it is hardly surprising that many of us go one step further and get haemorrhoids! Factors that favour congestion and enlargement of anal cushions relate principally to straining, either to initiate or complete a bowel action or in the process of heavy physical exertion, but also include such things as menstruation and pregnancy, where there is more generalized pelvic congestion.

To the best of my knowledge there is no proven connection between haemorrhoids and the development of varicose veins in the legs or between haemorrhoids and prolonged sitting on hard or cold surfaces. Individuals who have experienced these associations may not necessarily have had true haemorrhoids to start with. Haemorrhoids are frequently diagnosed in people complaining of painful perianal lumps that have little if anything to do with true haemorrhoids.

How can haemorrhoids be treated?

Make no mistake; haemorrhoids are not a life-threatening condition! Symptoms, even when present for years, are generally only of nuisance value. And having tolerated them for years, nearly everyone can keep them just a bit longer if they wish. But when bleeding, prolapse, and other symptoms finally become too much to bear, people bring in their haemorrhoids and ask for help!

The first thing to emphasize is that haemorrhoids are 'dynamic' structures. By this, I mean that they may vary in size and symptoms from day to day or from week to week. At some times they may be congested and produce prominent bleeding and prolapse. At other times they may be quite undetectable.

The commonly held notion of haemorrhoids as a 'bunch of grapes' suggests an all-or-nothing phenomenon. A more accurate analogy is that of one or more small sponges—prone to bleed and protrude when congested and swollen yet collapsed and unremarkable when not.

Fluctuations in the symptoms caused by haemorrhoids probably reflect subtle changes in our bowel habits. The more 'pressure' brought to bear on the upper anal canal, usually by a combination of straining and prolonged sitting on the toilet, the more likely haemorrhoids are to become engorged and to produce symptoms. The first step in treating our haemorrhoids is to make sure that both the total amount of time we spend on the toilet and the amount of straining required to effect a bowel action are kept to an absolute minimum.

In short, the first step in treating haemorrhoids is to establish an effective bowel habit, in which evacuation is easy both to initiate and to complete. This, of course, goes back to the seven elements of a highly effective bowel habit outlined in Chapter 2. Quick on and quick off! Although many haemorrhoids do require other treatments aimed at removing or shrinking them, recurrence of haemorrhoids is very much more likely if the underlying pattern of straining and prolonged sitting on the toilet is not corrected.

It is interesting to note that haemorrhoids are traditionally thought to be the result of constipation and that the adoption of a high fibre diet or a dietary fibre supplement is often the first step recommended for their treatment. Yet haemorrhoids are more commonly seen in men, who, as I've already said and who we all know, anyway, are much less prone to constipation than are women. If constipation were the main cause of haemorrhoids, surely there would be a massive predominance of women as sufferers!

In fact, men often have fast-moving bowels with soft, frequent, and even urgent bowel movements. Getting started is rarely a problem for men. But finishing off is often a problem and, as we know, men often spend a long time on the toilet trying to finish off—waiting and wiping, sitting and straining. Their 'total toilet time' is high and they often have to strain to complete evacuation. This represents a sure recipe for developing haemorrhoids.

Time and time again, doctors make the mistake of tackling haemorrhoids by surgery and other means—often involving quite painful treatments—without ever addressing the root cause (the poor underlying bowel habit) or taking steps to help prevent early recurrence. Time and time again, I have seen patients with long-standing symptoms of prolapse and bleeding 'cure' their symptoms by nothing more than a change in their pattern of going to the toilet. Fibre supplements are fine if your problem is a sluggish bowel habit; combining a solid stool and a strong urge is the way to go if you are struggling to complete evacuation (see Chapter 4).

Common and 'new' haemorrhoid treatments

Because haemorrhoidal symptoms are so common, because they are rarely serious, and because they often fluctuate of their own accord, this has proven a fertile field for 'new' treatments and outright quackery. Laser, infra-red, and cryotherapy (freezing) are just a few treatments that have come and gone (and come again!). This is a safe and lucrative area in which charlatans and 'technomaniacs' have been able to flourish. The promise of a painless cure lures unsuspecting haemorrhoids (and their owners) into expensive therapies that offer nothing more—and sometimes a whole lot less—than the time-honoured alternatives.

Injection of haemorrhoids (sclerotherapy)

By directly injecting the swollen haemorrhoid with a solution of oil and alcohol, haemorrhoids can be made to shrivel. This treatment is most applicable for control of bleeding but can also be used to treat some cases of prolapse. Because the surface of the haemorrhoid has no sensation, this treatment can be readily performed in a doctor's surgery without pain. Since it needs to be done through a short, broad, cylindrical instrument (called a proctoscope) placed in the anus, it is uncomfortable and undignified. Thankfully, this treatment is also very quick. Treatment is usually over in under five minutes.

Not uncommonly, this treatment is associated with some residual discomfort around the anus that might last two or three days. Rarely, there may be delayed bleeding from one or other injection site. This is a simple, cheap, and safe treatment for small to moderate haemorrhoids.

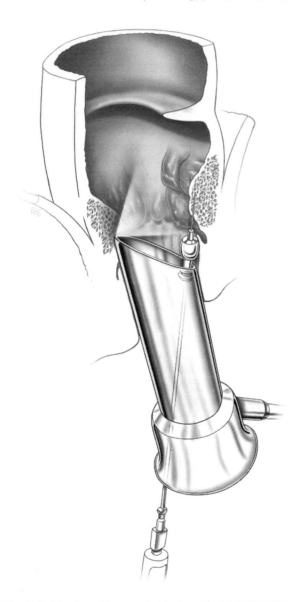

Fig. 5.2 Injection of haemorrhoids through a proctoscope can be easily performed in a doctor's surgery.

Banding of haemorrhoids

For larger haemorrhoids, where prolapse is a prominent complaint, tiny rubber bands can be placed at the base of the haemorrhoids using special instruments. This effectively 'strangles' the haemorrhoid and encourages it to shrivel. It is much like the process for castrating baby rams or bull calves!

Banding can also be readily performed in the doctor's surgery without undue pain or discomfort. This still requires the insertion of a proctoscope and it can produce some lingering discomfort. It takes very little time (again, usually under five minutes) and like injection treatment is very safe.

The good thing about both injection and banding—which can of course be used in combination—is that patients who have this treatment walk in and can generally walk out ten minutes later. Not all the haemorrhoids present need to be treated at the first sitting and treatment can be easily spread out over two or three visits. If treatment doesn't work well, little has been lost. If it only partly works, treatment can be repeated. And if symptoms go away only to recur months or years later, the chances are that banding or injection will be effective once again.

The down-side of injection and banding is that it doesn't always control the symptoms. Even if it does, recurrence is not infrequent, especially if an underlying problem with an ineffective bowel habit cannot be corrected.

Finally, for very large haemorrhoids, banding and injection are unlikely ever to be effective. Alas, for these poor sufferers, there are some haemorrhoids that simply cannot be controlled by anything other than surgery.

Haemorrhoidectomy

Haemorrhoidectomy involves the surgical removal of the haemorrhoids themselves along with the nearby skin and anal lining at that location. The more haemorrhoids that are present, the more tissue that needs to be removed. Once removed a large part of the underlying internal anal sphincter is exposed. Opening one's bowels after this

(a)

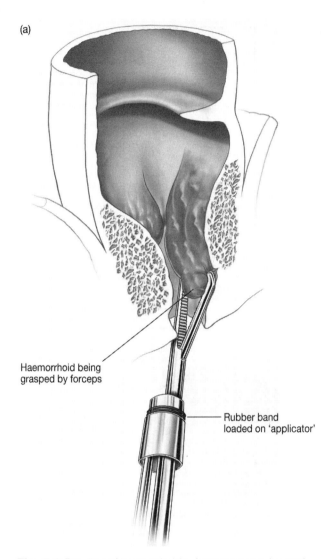

Haemorrhoid being
grasped by forceps

Rubber band
loaded on 'applicator'

Fig. 5.3 Banding of haemorrhoids. A proctoscope is used
but has not been shown in these illustrations.

(b)

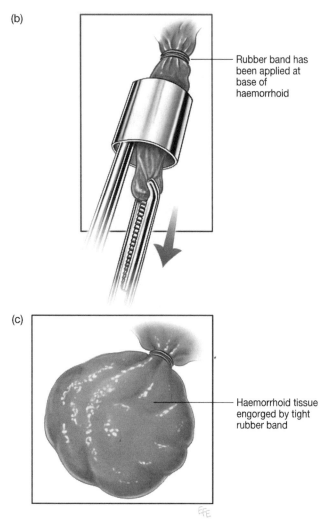

Rubber band has been applied at base of haemorrhoid

(c)

Haemorrhoid tissue engorged by tight rubber band

Fig. 5.3 (*Continued*)

operation can be very painful and haemorrhoidectomy has a well-deserved reputation for its ugly post-operative recovery period.

Nevertheless, haemorrhoidectomy remains the most predictably effective and long-lasting of all haemorrhoid treatments. Provided the post-operative period is managed with care and, above all, compassion, very few people are uncomfortable after about two weeks. And provided the haemorrhoids really did warrant surgery (many patients have been holding on to their piles for decades!), the end result is a grateful individual who wishes he or she had done this years before.

Here are some useful tips and warnings for those who have been advised to have a haemorrhoidectomy.

1. If you strain to open your bowels on a regular basis or if you spend a long time sitting on the toilet, you may find this to be an important and reversible cause for your haemorrhoids. More importantly, habitual straining before haemorrhoidectomy is a predictable recipe for misery in the post-operative period. The combination of a well-established pattern of straining on the toilet and the very painful anal wounds that follow haemorrhoidectomy makes the process of evacuating after haemorrhoidectomy diabolically painful. Please attend to your bowel habit (see Chapter 4) before proceeding. Even if your haemorrhoidal symptoms do not go away, you will at least make your post-operative recovery so much easier.

2. Ensure that your bowels are working freely leading up to your haemorrhoidectomy. This is one situation where a slightly faster moving stool may be a big help even if only for a short while. A gentle fibre supplement or a mild osmotic laxative syrup (see Chapter 4) can be started 24 to 48 hours before surgery. Your surgeon will almost always prescribe something similar for you in the post-operative period as well.

3. Getting your bowels open after haemorrhoidectomy is the big hurdle. The laxatives taken before and prescribed

after surgery will ensure a reasonably fast colonic transit. You should complement this after surgery by plenty of drinking, eating, and walking. Avoid the temptation to lie in bed—whether in hospital or at home. Physical activity is an important stimulus for normal bowel contraction; prolonged rest in bed might slow things down.

4. After haemorrhoidectomy you may feel under some pressure to get your bowels open sooner rather than later, particularly as many surgeons will advise their patients to go home only after the first bowel action. Equally, nursing staff are anxious to see their patients through this important hurdle. The trouble is, if you try to evacuate in advance of a genuinely powerful urge (that is, you engage in speculative visits to the toilet) you will be confronting the dual obstacles of an indifferent urge and an anal sphincter that is stubbornly but understandably reluctant to relax. This conflict between brain('I know I'm supposed to go') and anus ('I'm not letting anything through here!') lies at the very heart of post-haemorrhoidectomy grief.

So do not attempt to evacuate your bowels unless the urge is frankly critical, even if this needs to be induced artificially with an enema. Your surgeon will know only too well when to advise that an enema be given, if appropriate.

5. An important early complication of haemorrhoidectomy, not surprisingly, is failure to evacuate the rectum fully. This can result in a progressive build-up of faeces within the rectum, which we term **faecal impaction**. The impacted ball of faeces stretches the rectum and becomes frankly impossible to pass. Softer material then trickles around the solid ball and may ooze out without control (overflow incontinence). Enemas and even disimpaction under anaesthetic may be necessary to correct the problem.

Constant rectal pain, the sensation of rectal fullness, and overflow incontinence of soft faeces are sure signs of post-haemorrhoidectomy faecal impaction and must not be ignored. Luckily, the warning signs are simple. Human beings are very sensitive to any residue within the rectum.

If we have not completely emptied our bowels we generally sense this. After haemorrhoidectomy, failure to empty the rectum should be reported to your surgeon. If this fails to be resolved within 24 hours an enema should be administered to ensure complete rectal evacuation.

6. The other significant and avoidable complication of haemorrhoidectomy is healing of the wounds with narrowing or stricture formation. The best way to prevent the anal wounds from 'closing in' is to ensure the regular passage of a bulky though soft bowel action. This means that the healing anus is gently stretched by each action. To ensure that healing happens in this manner, I strongly recommend that you take a daily fibre supplement for a full four weeks after haemorrhoidectomy. At your follow-up examination, your surgeon will examine the anal canal to ensure that healing has proceeded without stricture formation.

Painless haemorrhoidectomy

Many people have claimed to perform haemorrhoidectomy without pain. To date, none of these techniques has stood the test of time! A relatively recent development, however, is the use of a stapling instrument that removes most (not all) of the haemorrhoidal material but does not leave behind any open wounds. It does, however, leave behind a complete circle of metal staples which remains indefinitely.

This technique is still relatively new but may prove a useful alternative to injection, banding, or haemorrhoidectomy. Your family doctor may not be aware of the procedure but will know of a specialist colorectal surgeon who can explain it to you in more detail. Stapled haemorrhoidectomy may prove to have a useful part to play in the treatment of haemorrhoids, but it is not going to be the solution for every haemorrhoid sufferer!

When haemorrhoids turn 'nasty'

No, haemorrhoids do not become cancerous! But they can cause trouble that has more than just 'nuisance value'.

Haemorrhoids can bleed to such an extent, usually over many, many months, as to cause anaemia. Anaemia results in a shortage of the oxygen-carrying haemoglobin within the bloodstream making the sufferer pale, lethargic, easily tired, and even short of breath; it can be detected by a simple blood test. Since anaemia can be due to many different causes, your doctor will need to test you extensively. But if your haemorrhoids are the cause of your anaemia they undoubtedly require treatment and, almost always, this means haemorrhoidectomy.

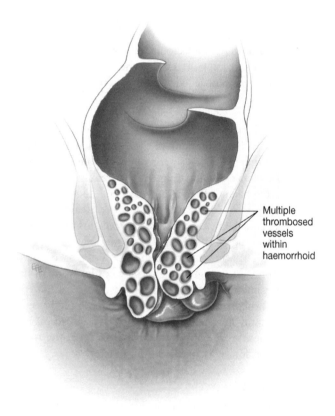

Multiple thrombosed vessels within haemorrhoid

Fig. 5.4 Painful prolapsed, thrombosed haemorrhoids.

In addition, haemorrhoids that have been bleeding and prolapsing for months or years can undergo painful thrombosis or clotting. This produces quite intense pain with one or more tender lumps present around the anus. It may take up to two weeks for the pain to subside while the lumps may take many weeks longer. Since haemorrhoids remain an ongoing problem in such cases long after the episode of thrombosis has finished, early haemorrhoidectomy is often a good way of treating not only the short-term pain and swelling, but also the longer-term problems of bleeding and prolapse.

* * * * *

Haemorrhoids are very common and do not usually cause enough trouble to warrant any action. From time to time, however, bleeding, prolapse, or thrombosis bring them out into the open. When clearly necessary, haemorrhoid treatment is generally successful and greatly appreciated.

Anal thrombosis

You now know that haemorrhoids can undergo thrombosis and can produce sudden pain and tender perianal lumps. Surprisingly few people, however, know that thrombosis of superficial blood vessels around the outer anal verge, rather than affecting the haemorrhoids themselves up at the anorectal junction, is at least ten times more frequent. Nearly everybody can recall at least one such episode of sudden pain and swelling, generally describing it as 'an attack of piles'.

Both superficial and true haemorrhoidal thromboses cause sudden pain and swelling. Many doctors group all of these conditions together and call them 'thrombosed haemorrhoids', but the majority of cases have nothing to do with true haemorrhoids and a better description would be **external anal thrombosis**.

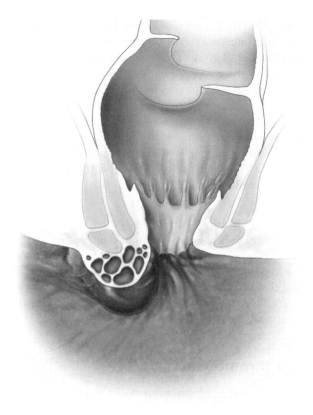

Fig. 5.5 A nasty but entirely external anal thrombosis. Compare this with the prolapsed, thrombosed haemorrhoids in Fig. 5.4.

What causes external thrombosis?

It goes without saying that blood should not normally clot spontaneously within our own blood vessels! However, if blood flow through any blood vessel—even the small ones under the perianal skin—becomes turbulent for any reason, spontaneous clotting can occur.

The usual factors that provoke anal thrombosis are all related to straining. Straining to deliver a baby is perhaps the number one cause—many women who have had no anal or bowel problems whatsoever during their pregnancy can still experience painful but entirely external anal thrombosis in the last stages of pregnancy, during, or just after delivery. Other common precipitating events include episodes of diarrhoea—anal thrombosis often complicates a bout of gastroenteritis—as well as vigorous physical exercise, especially involving the lifting of heavy objects.

The good news is that both external anal and haemorrhoidal thromboses always settle down by themselves. The pain can take up to two weeks to go away in extensive cases and the swelling several weeks longer. In the meantime, thromboses can discharge old blood clot, which can be a frightening development even though this is not at all dangerous.

Finally, although these thromboses always resolve of their own accord, they may leave behind a small residual skin tag as a kind of memento or souvenir of this painful episode, marking the spot where the mischief took place.

What should be done for external anal thrombosis?

Since these episodes always get better by themselves there is no absolute need to do anything about them. Painkillers and ice packs interspersed with hot baths and lots of sympathy will generally get you through.

Just the same, some episodes are so painful as to make it impossible even to think about doing anything else. Sadly, because this is a bottom problem it can be hard to find anyone to take you seriously. And you may not even be prepared to let your own doctor look at it! But it might be possible to have your anal thrombosis diagnosed and treated under local anaesthetic in just one brief visit to your doctor or, if not, a colorectal surgeon.

When I see individuals with an external anal thrombosis, I ask myself this simple question: 'Has this episode passed its worst?' In other words, if the pain is already subsiding then I do not believe that removing the thrombosis is likely to help abbreviate further the overall period of pain and disability. If, on the other hand, I see the thrombosis early on in its course while the pain is still at its worst, removing the thrombosis (usually under local anaesthetic but occasionally under general anaesthetic) is worthwhile.

A few final warnings about surgery for anal thrombosis

1. Except for the smallest of external thromboses, incising or 'nicking' the overlying skin to release the clot should not be done. In other words, once the thrombosis has reached a reasonable size—say anything over about eight to ten millimetres or half an inch long—it cannot be dealt with properly by just nicking the skin and trying to squeeze out the blood clot. Much better actually to remove the clot and overlying skin all in one.

2. Removing the thrombosis in this way leaves behind a small, open wound. This is rarely very painful but it will weep and ooze—like any raw skin surface—and it will require regular bathing to keep it clean. Wounds such as this can take four weeks or longer to heal completely.

3. The one instance in which I carefully recommend *against* removing anal thromboses is in women who have just delivered a baby. After a vaginal delivery, the pelvic floor is often swollen and stretched, and bowel function further affected by painkillers and stress (see Chapter 10). Adding a painful anal wound to this difficult combination makes for an even more grizzly recovery! This applies equally to true prolapsed thrombosed haemorrhoids in women who have just delivered babies.

Put simply, anal and haemorrhoidal thromboses that occur after vaginal delivery are better left to subside by themselves. By all means get your bottom examined by a specialist but don't rush into anal surgery too soon after delivery.

Other causes of prolapse

Haemorrhoids are not the only things that can prolapse and protrude from the anal canal. Three other things to bear in mind are:

1. Anal canal polyps

These are firm, pale, fibrous polyps arising form about halfway up the anal canal (Figure 5.6). They are a bit like an internal version of a perianal skin tag. They arise in response to nearby trouble—haemorrhoids above, or anal fissure below—but they are themselves quite harmless. Anal canal polyps do not transform into true tumours although if they become large enough to prolapse (usually after a bowel action) they can cause concern and become a general nuisance. They are readily removed surgically under light general anaesthesia.

2. Rectal polyps

A large rectal polyp is almost always a true tumour. Most are bengin—that is, not a cancer—but they do have the potential to transform into cancer if ignored for many months or years. Rectal polyps that are situated low down in the rectum or that have grown on a long stalk may protrude from the anus, again usually after having a bowel action (Figure 5.7). The surface of these polyps is prone to bleed if touched or traumatized. Similarly, the polyp surface tends to produce excess mucus. As a result, bleeding and blood-stained mucus are common symptoms accompanying a prolapsing rectal polyp.

Never forget, rectal bleeding is a cardinal symptom of rectal tumours, both benign and cancerous, and must never be ignored. Rectal bleeding must always be assessed by your doctor, especially if there is associated prolapse.

3. Rectal prolapse

In some circumstances the entire circumference of the rectum can slide down and turn in on itself to protrude

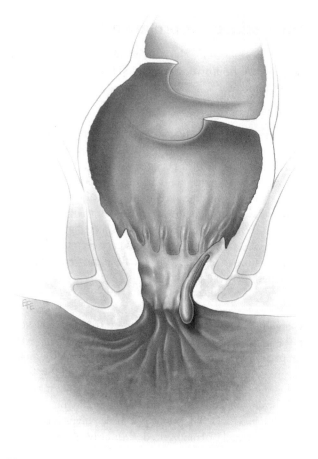

Fig. 5.6 Prolapsing, fibrous polyp of the anal canal.

from the anal canal. This may involve only the superficial lining of the rectal wall—called **rectal mucosal** prolapse. In more advanced cases, the entire thickness of the rectal wall prolapses—this is called **full thickness prolapse**. Both kinds of rectal prolapse are also most likely to be noticed after a bowel action but may also be provoked by

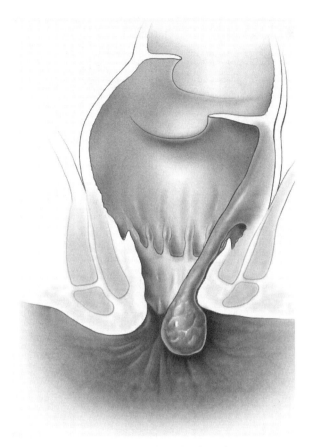

Fig. 5.7 Rectal polyp on a stalk prolapsing after a bowel action.

squatting and straining, and may even be permanently prolapsed in extreme cases.

Minor mucosal rectal prolapse looks like and produces symptoms very similar to haemorrhoids. These include bright red bleeding, protrusion, and mucus discharge. Full thickness prolapse also produces these symptoms but it is noticeably more bulky.

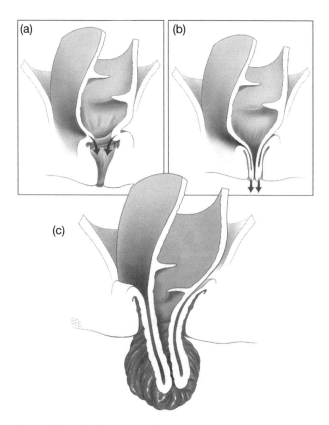

Fig. 5.8 Full thickness rectal prolapse.

With repeated full thickness prolapse, the anal sphincter muscles can become stretched and are prone to become weakened. This can lead to problems with continence, initially to gas but subsequently even to stool. Rectal prolapse is one of very few potentially reversible causes of anal sphincter weakness and is an important condition to identify and correct in people complaining of incontinence of flatus or faeces.

Rarely, full thickness rectal prolapse can become trapped in its prolapsed position ('incarcerated') and have its blood supply compressed ('strangulated'). This is a painful and urgent situation which requires the immediate attention of an expert in this field. Usually the prolapse can be returned (called 'reduced' in medical terms) after the individual has been given strong analgesics and sometimes even after a light anaesthetic. The prolapse must then be corrected at the earliest opportunity.

What causes rectal prolapse?

Minor mucosal prolapse is most commonly seen in the elderly and especially in elderly women. It is best thought of as an age-related 'weakness', a bit like the hem falling from a well-worn skirt or dress. Minor prolapse may also be aggravated by excessive straining on the toilet and where mucosal prolapse does occur in younger people, straining is often a significant cause.

On the other hand full thickness rectal prolapse can appear in both males and females and at all ages from infancy to old age. It is seen in women who have never had children as well as in those who have had many. Many theories to explain the occurrence of full thickness rectal prolapse have been proposed. Whilst it goes without saying that there must be weakness of the structures that support the rectum and hold it in its usual position, there is no generally agreed explanation as to why this weakness occurs.

How is rectal prolapse treated?

Mucosal prolapse is treated much the same as are haemorrhoids. This ranges from no treatment at all—the prolapse is, after all, of 'nuisance value' only—to injection sclerotherapy, rubber band ligation, and even surgical excision resembling haemorrhoidectomy. The results are generally very good although further prolapse can always occur. Sometimes mucosal prolapse is treated successfully only to see the patient return after months or years with a more established full thickness rectal prolapse.

Most people suffering from full thickness rectal prolapse want it fixed. The discomfort of the prolapse, the
bleeding and mucus discharge, and the interference with
continence can make life miserable. And the solution
always involves surgery. Over the years many different
operations have been developed for this condition and
many of these operations are still in practice. You should
be assessed by a specialist surgeon with particular expert-
ise in the treatment of rectal prolapse who will be able to
advise you of the most appropriate procedure in your case.

In simple terms, however, there are two basic
approaches to surgical repair of rectal prolapse—either
from below or via the abdomen.

1. From below

Operations to correct rectal prolapse that are performed
through the anus itself have the advantage of being less
traumatic and, therefore, safer in the elderly and frail.
Recurrence of the prolapse, however, is more common
than with techniques using an abdominal approach. If
recurrence does occur, the same anal procedure may be
repeated; alternatively, an abdominal approach may then
be considered more appropriate.

2. Via the abdomen

The use of an abdominal incision—even if using keyhole
surgery—turns this approach into a more major undertaking. It is generally preferred in younger patients and in
those with the most extensive degrees of rectal prolapse.
Because these techniques all involve dissection close to
the nerves that supply sexual function in men, this is not
usually the first surgical option in men with rectal prolapse. Once again the advice of a surgeon expert in this
area is vital.

Anal fissure

An anal fissure is a split or tear in the lining of the
lowest part of the anal canal. It is usually no more than

5 mm (less than a quarter of a inch) long and 2 or 3 mm deep. But it can cause terrible anal pain and can make life utterly miserable.

Characteristically, people who have an anal fissure find that pain is provoked by having their bowels open. The passage of stool literally splits the fissure open causing a tearing pain and, not infrequently, some fresh bleeding seen on the toilet paper. Aching and throbbing around the anus can then last for hours after each bowel action. Patients with anal fissure literally dread the prospect of having their bowels open; if this describes your symptoms, the chances are very high that you have an anal fissure.

What causes anal fissure?

There are two commonly recorded precipitating events: passage of a constipated bowel motion and delivering a baby. It isn't too difficult to understand how the passage of a big, hard bowel motion can split the anus. But how a vaginal delivery does this is not so clear. In either event, this small and shallow anal wound causes a large amount of trouble.

Sometimes anal fissures heal of their own accord never to reappear. This is referred to as an acute anal fissure. Often, however, they recur and heal only to recur again or they become a permanent feature causing intractable symptoms. These are called chronic anal fissures and without treatment they will never go away. The presence of a tender, slightly swollen skin tag at the outer margin of the fissure is a good sign that the anal fissure has become chronic.

How can anal fissure be treated?

Like haemorrhoids, anal fissure is not a dangerous condition and the need for treatment is generally determined by just how much pain and bother the fissure is causing. Some people are content to know that there isn't anything seriously wrong with them and leave it at that.

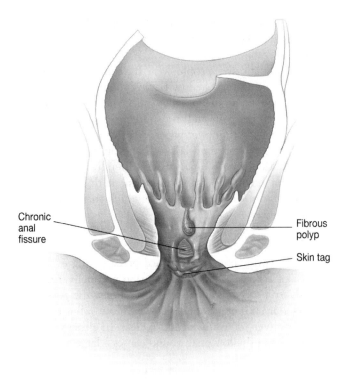

Chronic anal fissure

Fibrous polyp

Skin tag

Fig. 5.9 A chronic anal fissure with 'sentinel' skin tag and fibrous anal canal polyp (another common feature).

Most, however, are greatly inconvenienced by the fissure and request active assistance.

Over many years surgeons have come to recognize that the answer to treating an anal fissure is not to be found in cutting out the fissure itself. Rather, the underlying fault seems to be overactivity of the internal anal sphincter muscle. This helps to explain why, when the bottom end in question is examined, the anus appears to be held so tightly clamped. It also helps explain why such a small wound will not heal when much larger ones left after some anal operations (haemorrhoidectomy, for example) seem to heal so readily.

In other words, to treat anal fissure we have to disable the internal anal sphincter. If we can get the internal anal sphincter to relax, the pain and bleeding will subside and the anal fissure will actually heal. There are numerous ways that the internal anal sphincter can be made to relax. These are the currently available treatments for anal fissure.

1. Glyceryl trinitrate (GTN) cream

When applied directly to the skin of the lower anal canal and just inside the anal verge, GTN cream releases a chemical that causes the internal anal sphincter to relax. This is not enough to result in problems with continence but it is usually sufficient to give relief from both pain and bleeding. A common side-effect is headache or even a degree of light-headedness; sometimes these side-effects make it impossible to continue with treatment.

There are conflicting reports of just how many people are actually cured by GTN cream. If the cream is going to have any chance at all it should be used for six to eight weeks or longer. Even so, in my experience, complete and lasting healing of the fissure is infrequent, perhaps in about a quarter of those who start treatment. Most people recognize that even if they are much more comfortable when using the cream, their bottoms are not 'one hundred per cent'. Pain and bleeding rapidly return once the treatment is stopped. To the best of current knowledge, there is no reason not to continue GTN indefinitely if you wish. Even if you have decided to proceed to other treatment—surgery, for example—you can continue to use GTN cream to control symptoms right up until your surgery is performed.

2. Nifedipine, Diltiazem

These drugs—part of the family of drugs called 'calcium channel blockers' and usually used in the treatment of high blood pressure and other cardiovascular conditions—have been shown to be effective both as a cream applied like GTN cream or in oral (tablet) form. They don't appear to be any more effective than GTN cream and can also cause troublesome side-effects (headaches, flushing) but they might help in some cases where GTN did not.

3. 'Botox'

This is short for botulinum toxin. That's right, the toxin that causes the muscle spasm and paralysis of botulism! It is not, however the actual organism that is responsible for this serious infection, so injecting the botox into the internal anal sphincter does not cause botulism. It does, however, relax the internal anal sphincter enough to permit healing of chronic anal fissure in many cases and, it seems, with very few side-effects. Botox is not, however, readily available and the injection of this notionally noxious agent is not yet in widespread use.

4. Surgery

Surgery provides the most reliable and long-lasting means of interfering with internal anal sphincter function. A forcible stretch of the anus—obviously under appropriate anaesthetic—damages the internal anal sphincter and allows the fissure to heal. Unfortunately, it is difficult to gauge just how far to stretch the anus and overdoing the stretch can result in permanent incontinence, usually of gas.

As a result, surgeons have modified this operation to involve a simple cut of the lower margin of the internal anal sphincter. This is called 'sphincterotomy' and can be performed under either general or local anaesthetic. Sphincterotomy preserves normal function in the upper half to two-thirds of the anal sphincter and reduces the risk of permanent problems with control over gas to about 5 per cent (1 in 20 cases). The more cautious the surgeon, the less likely is incontinence to occur. Of course, long-term cure may also be less likely if the surgeon is too cautious when cutting the internal anal sphincter!

For all this talk about sphincterotomy causing incontinence, many people with anal fissure still choose—or frankly need—this operation for long-term cure. Your doctor will be able to guide you through the various treatment alternatives.

Perianal abscess

Perianal infection is a common occurrence. This is hardly surprising—it has been estimated that about half the weight of human faeces is made up of bacteria alone! With all those bugs passing through the anus every day, sooner or later some of them are going to get into the wrong spot. In fact, it is amazing that infection around the anus isn't more common!

Most perianal abscesses begin when bacteria find their way into the anal crypt glands (see Fig. 5.10). These little mucus-producing glands are located between internal and external anal sphincter muscles about halfway up the anal canal. Each of us has approximately ten to twelve crypt glands spread around the anal canal at its mid-level. Once the bacteria enter the gland, they multiply rapidly and an abscess develops in the tight space between the two sphincter muscles. As more and more pus forms, this forces its way between the muscles down towards the perianal skin or sometimes out and away from the anal canal, between bundles of external anal sphincter muscles. Rarely, pus will force its way upwards between the two sphincter muscles settling above the sphincter and forming an abscess around the rectum.

Perianal abscesses usually produce pain around the anus that develops over a matter of days. There may be fever and loss of appetite as well as a general sense of being unwell. As the abscess increases in size and reaches the perianal skin, there is obvious local infection: redness, swelling, and a tender firmness directly over the abscess. These features make perianal abscesses easily distinguishable from other causes of perianal pain such as anal fissure and thrombosis. The abscess can 'point' at any position around the anus, front or back, left or right.

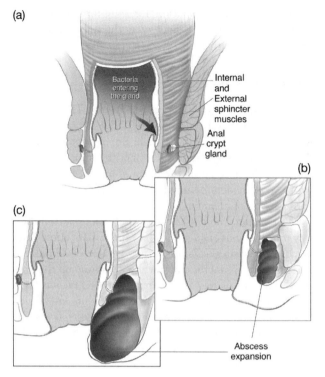

(a)

Bacteria entering the gland

Internal and External sphincter muscles

Anal crypt gland

(b)

(c)

Abscess expansion

Fig. 5.10 Perianal abscesses start as an infection in the anal crypt gland, which expands between or through the anal sphincters to reach the surface around the anal opening.

Like abscesses elsewhere in the body, perianal abscesses generally build up to a 'head' and can spontaneously burst through the skin, relieving the tension. Often, however, they are so painful in the phase leading up to spontaneous rupture that surgery is needed to speed up this process. The abscess can be readily drained under anaesthetic to release the pus and control the pain.

Unfortunately, this is not usually the end of the story! Most perianal abscesses have a narrow communication with the anal canal. This is, of course, where the bacteria originally found their way into the crypt gland and this point of entry frequently remains open. It acts as an ongoing source of infection so that while the drainage point might gradually heal, infection often builds up again. Rather than form another full-blown abscess, however, it is more common for infection to build up intermittently and discharge—pus, blood, and even some faecal particles—from the external drainage point. This condition is called **anal fistula** and it is a frequent development after a perianal abscess has either burst spontaneously or has been drained by your doctor (Figure 5.11).

Draining a perianal abscess, even a large one, is simple in both principle and practice. On the other hand, dealing with the underlying fistula—the communication with the anal canal—is not. This is because surgery for anal fistula often involves cutting some of the sphincter muscle. Luckily, human anal sphincters have plenty in reserve and can be partially cut without undue concern about the development of incontinence. But the sphincter muscle should never be cut indiscriminately and surgery for fistula should always be performed by a specialist experienced in this area.

Perianal abscess is common, easily diagnosed, and simply treated. The underlying fistula, however, causes repeated infections and should be assessed and treated by an expert.

Skin tags

The perianal skin has a very limited repertoire! In response to most anal conditions, the perianal skin tends to form a skin tag. Haemorrhoids and anal fissure may be associated with skin tags that can remain long after the haemorrhoid or fissure has gone. Anal thrombosis may also subside and leave behind one or more skin tags. Other anal diseases—notably Crohn's disease (see Chapter 9)—are also often accompanied by skin tag formation.

Skin tags can be single or multiple and can assume a wide range of shapes and sizes. They are frequently

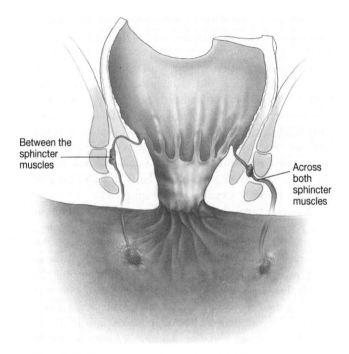

Between the sphincter muscles

Across both sphincter muscles

Fig. 5.11 Two common types of anal fistula.

misdiagnosed as haemorrhoids or referred to as 'piles', but are, of course, nothing more than excess folds of skin. They either point to the fact that some other anal problem currently exists or serve as souvenirs of previous anal mischief.

Skin tags are rarely the root cause of perianal symptoms.

When they are associated with pain, think of anal fissure.

When they are associated with painless bleeding, think of underlying haemorrhoids.

When they are associated with difficulty wiping up after a bowel action, think of pursuing a firmer bowel motion. This is the most common reason why people are referred to me to have their skin tags excised, but the skin tags themselves rarely have anything at all to do with people's difficulty in maintaining the perianal skin in a clean and dry state. The problem for these individuals is almost always an excessively soft stool consistency making completion of evacuation impossible. The solution does not lie with excision of the skin tag!

Skin tags can be excised if they are 'getting in the way' or causing cosmetic problems. But be warned, recovery after excision of skin tags can be painful and may leave behind one or more raw surfaces that require regular bathing. This reinforces the point that skin tags should not be removed just because they are there. Make sure the associated anal problems (fissure, haemorrhoids, soiling, etc.) are corrected first. Very often, the skin tags can then be comfortably left alone for good.

Pelvic floor strain

As a bowel diseases specialist, I am regularly asked to see people with intractable or unresponsive perianal pain. Fissure, abscesses, and thromboses have all long been excluded. Cancer and Crohn's disease have been ruled out. Trials of treatment with antibiotics or anal operations such as haemorrhoidectomy or sphincterotomy, performed in desperation, have failed.

An important cause of intractable perianal pain, however, is not described in text books or even in the recent scientific literature. It has no long-established or widely accepted name. I call this **pelvic floor strain**, since it appears to arise from the muscles and bony prominences of the pelvic floor and since it is readily aggravated by certain physical factors.

A typical case will describe the following:

1. Pain is felt around the anus, not at the skin level but a few centimetres inside. It may be felt in front of the anus and men may describe it as being under the base of the scrotum. Often it is clearly worse on one side (left or right) than the other.

2. Pain is generally at its lowest point after a night's sleep and tends to deteriorate as the day wears on, especially if the

individual has had to spend a long time on his or her feet or has been exercising vigorously. Step climbing and bicycle riding are particularly likely to aggravate pelvic floor strain.

3. Sitting for prolonged periods, especially on hard sur-faces, is another frequent aggravating factor. Sufferers describe having to shift regularly in their seats to lift one buttock off the chair literally to 'give it a rest'. Another description used is a sensation of sitting on a lump like having a tennis ball under their bottom.

4. Even having a bowel action can trigger the pain. The pelvic floor has a well-defined 'hole' through which the anus passes. As stool passes through this opening in the pelvic floor it may stretch the muscle at this point and provoke pain from these abnormally sensitive structures. The pain provoked by a bowel action may last for a num-ber of hours and this pattern may cause the condition to be confused with anal fissure. Similarly, sexual intercourse may provoke this pain in women for precisely the same reasons since penetration makes direct contact with the structures of the pelvic floor.

5. Examining the tail end of someone with pelvic floor strain usually clinches the diagnosis. Fissure, abscesses, and thromboses are readily excluded. Gentle prodding through the skin around the anus allows the examining doctor to put pressure over the bony prominences of the pelvic floor. These can also be touched more directly during careful internal rectal examination. Almost invariably, one or more points of exquisite bony or muscular tenderness can be found and the examination itself characteristically trig-gers or worsens the pain. After a thorough examination, there is rarely any doubt as to the diagnosis!

What causes pelvic floor strain?

I'm afraid I don't know the answer to this. In some people it can be traced back to a distinct event such as lifting a heavy object or digging a deep trench. It may relate to a recent change in physical exercise such as having started bicycle riding or jogging. This reinforces the concept of a muscle strain, a bit like a sporting injury.

In others, however, pelvic floor strain just seems to have developed over months or years and it behaves a little more like chronic arthritis, improving and deteriorating unpredictably. Whatever the cause, pelvic floor strain tends to run its own course and sufferers must learn to accept and live with it as best they can.

Can anything be done to treat pelvic floor strain?

Definitely yes! The basic steps and treatment are:

1. *Cushions and pillows* to reduce direct pressure when sitting for lengthy periods. Some people prefer doughnut shaped cushions; others do not.

2. *Modify your physical exercise.* Avoid aggravating your pelvic floor strain by bicycle riding, step climbing, jogging, etc.; if possible, do more exercise in a swimming pool where the water takes some of the weight off your pelvic floor.

3. *Avoid straining at stool.* Easy evacuation of formed stools should minimize the tendency for passage of stool to trigger your pain.

4. *Anti-inflammatory painkillers* are the most active medicines in pelvic floor strain. Since they don't actually fix the problem, they needn't be taken every day, only when symptoms are bad. You should consult your own doctor for the best advice on which anti-inflammatory agent would be most suitable for you.

5. *Physiotherapy.* Exercising a painful pelvic floor generally only aggravates the pain of pelvic floor strain. Pelvic floor exercises—a bit like dietary fibre—have become something of a 'cure all' for pelvic floor problems, especially in women. But this is most definitely one area in which pelvic floor exercises are *not* advisable. Rest, not exercise, is the key!

On the other hand, physiotherapists—and especially those with an interest in pelvic floor problems—may be

able to help with treatment such as ultrasound and inter-
ferential. Your family doctor can help direct you to an
appropriately trained physiotherapist in your area.

Proctalgia

Sudden, short-lived perianal, and perirectal pain is common. In fact I don't know a single person who hasn't
experienced it at some stage or other! Naturally it can be
of varying intensity and duration. Patients of mine have
described episodes of sufficient severity to cause them to
faint! Commonly, sufferers are unable even to move for
the brief duration of the attack. It can also occur with
varying frequency, an exceedingly rare event in many of
us but an almost daily occurrence in others.

Although we immediately assume that the pain is coming from the anus or lower rectum, it is almost certainly
coming from the muscles immediately surrounding this
point. These are the muscles of the pelvic floor and the
puborectalis muscle in particular. Cramp or spasm of this
muscle—just like that occurring in other muscles such as
in the calf—is thought to explain what we call **proctalgia**.

It is not at all clear why this muscle suddenly goes into
spasm and why some people are more prone to suffer from
this than are others. Some believe that it is a bit like a
tension headache, occurring at times of stress or in highly
stressed individuals. Regardless, it is usually so fleeting—
lasting literally a matter of seconds—and so infrequent
that it rarely causes sufficient bother even to bring to the
attention of your doctor.

For those of you who find that proctalgia starts to
become more of a bother, or even a recurring nightmare
of severe pain appearing out of the blue, there are some
simple steps that may be of help.

1. *Heat* is a useful muscle relaxant. The simple act of sitting
on a heat pad or a hot water bottle, or taking a hot bath
may be beneficial during a more long-lasting episode. An
inflammatory painkiller may also be effective. The problem

is that episodes of proctalgia are often so short-lived that they wear off and disappear well before the bath is poured or the medication is properly absorbed!

2. *Anti-inflammatory medication* can also be taken in suppository form. Yet absorption of the drug is no faster when given by suppository than when taken by tablet. On the other hand, the simple act of inserting the suppository might release the cramp by stretching the puborectalis muscle, not unlike pulling back on the toes and foot to stretch a cramped calf muscle. The relief gained from inserting a suppository might be noticed almost immediately, making insertion of anti-inflammatory suppositories an especially useful strategy for occasional, severe attacks.

For those of you who experience proctalgia on a daily or nightly basis (evening is said to be a common time for attacks to occur), regular anti-inflammatory medication might be helpful. Some doctors also recommend the popular and traditional anti-spasmodic medication Quinine for people whose proctalgia is frequent.

A careful examination by a doctor will exclude other more serious or more readily correctable causes for your pain. The reassurance that there is no sinister underlying problem and some simple strategies for dealing with severe or recurring bouts of pain are the only treatment that is generally required.

6
Itching and burning
(pruritus ani)

and it burns, burns, burns, the ring of fire …

Johnny Cash

An itching, burning, stinging bottom is an almost universal experience. For most people it is only an occasional problem; for many others, however, it is a recurring or constant nightmare. No other symptom—not even pain—is more distressing, more infuriating, or ultimately more exhausting. The need to scratch your bottom can be intense, driving you into the nearest toilet to get a little privacy or leaving you open to ridicule if seen scratching in public!

With scratching, the perianal skin becomes broken. This produces some spotting of blood as well as the weeping that inevitably occurs from any raw area of skin. This moisture further damages the surface barrier of the perianal skin leading to damp, pale, thickened skin with areas of splitting or even shallow ulceration. Burning pain and a stinging sensation when the skin comes in contact with hot water (in the shower, for example) add to the misery.

As a measure of how frequent this problem is, just note how many creams and ointments are available to help control these symptoms. Proctesedyl, Scheriproct, Ultraproct, Rectinol, and Anusol … the list goes on! And as a measure of just how distressing these symptoms are, take note of the cost of these preparations and the expense to which people are prepared to go to seek relief. But, at best, these creams only treat the symptoms, numbing the skin with dilute local anaesthetic or promoting healing of ulcerated skin with low dose steroids. The root cause is not addressed and the itching and burning almost always recur.

What causes perianal itch?

There are a number of different causes of pruritus ani.

In children, especially, pinworms are a well-known cause. Simple inspection of the perianal skin is usually sufficient to see the worms and to make the diagnosis. The whole family should be treated to safeguard against re-infection.

Certain skin diseases—psoriasis and eczema, for example—can also affect the perianal skin. The perianal skin, however, is rarely affected on its own. A history of these skin conditions affecting other more usual sites generally makes it easy to make the diagnosis and prescribe appropriate treatment.

Contact dermatitis is an allergic or hypersensitivity reaction to chemicals coming in contact with perianal skin. Ironically, the list of 'culprits' includes many of the creams prescribed for perianal use listed above, the local anaesthetic component in particular being prone to provoke a reaction. Once the offending chemical is withdrawn the dermatitis should subside.

Fungal infections can also cause pruritus ani. Such infections tend to cause a well-defined, red rash with a scaly, slightly raised outer margin. Scrapings of skin from the rash can be sent for culture in the laboratory to make the diagnosis. Unfortunately, steroid creams do calm the red angry element of the rash but do not in any way eradicate the fungal infection! Once the steroid cream is stopped, the rash and itching return.

If a fungal infection is confirmed—or even if it is just strongly suspected on the basis of the appearance of the rash—anti-fungal creams should be used. Your doctor or your pharmacist will be able to advise on the best choice of cream. Unlike most antibiotics, however, many anti-fungal creams need to be applied regularly over three to four weeks to eradicate the fungus completely.

In addition, fungi can often survive standard machine washing. This means that contaminated underwear may not be completely cleaned in the wash. About one week after commencing anti-fungal cream, you might like to put your underwear in a pot of boiling water and leave them there for 20 minutes. Alternatively, it might be a good opportunity to throw out your old underwear and buy some new ones.

If fungal infection recurs despite this treatment, you may need to eradicate fungus completely from your gastrointestinal tract with anti-fungal tablets. You may also need to consider some dietary modification—again, your doctor or even a dietician should be consulted.

Having talked about all these different causes of an itchy bottom, the truth remains that well over 90 per cent of the cases of pruritus ani that I see do not fit into any of these groups. In fact, the vast majority of adults with this complaint have what I call **common or garden variety pruritus ani**.

Some important and characteristic features of this common complaint are:

1. This is a predominantly (but not exclusively) male problem.

2. Symptoms are generally worst immediately after a bowel action and at night time or, less often, immediately before a bowel action.

3. Exercise and perspiration may also aggravate symptoms.

For all the grief caused by intractable pruritus ani, despite all the various creams, lotions, and powders applied, and even though specialist consultation is often needed, the underlying cause of common or garden variety pruritus ani is terribly simple. If the perianal skin is allowed to get moist or soiled or both, it will be prone to itching. If the perianal skin is kept clean and dry, it will not.

This does not mean that people with pruritus ani are 'dirty' or unhygienic. In fact, many sufferers are meticulous—overly so in some instances—about washing and cleaning their tail ends. Yet when I examine them in my surgery, a gentle wipe with gauze over the anal verge will often reveal the culprits: particles of soft faeces that have trickled out onto the perianal skin.

The perianal skin is surprisingly sensitive to the constant presence of particulate faecal matter. It is one thing to have a formed stool pass through the anus and across the perianal skin once or twice a day. It is quite another to have soft, moist faecal material in constant contact with this skin!

Does this mean that people with pruritus ani have a deficient anal sphincter mechanism? No, it does not. In Chapter 3, I described the pattern of passive soiling of soft stool, the characteristic pattern of faecal incontinence in men. In many respects common or garden variety pruritus ani—which is also a predominantly male problem—is a variant of this passive incontinence. This also explains why the itching is often worse just after a bowel action and why burning discomfort may occur during exercise. It also points fairly and squarely to soft stool as the root cause.

The first and most important step in bringing pruritus ani under control is to establish and then maintain a solid stool consistency. This will enable more complete rectal emptying, making it much less likely for any faecal matter to seep out after a bowel action. In the process of modifying the diet to get your bowel habit more solid, you will also reduce gas production. By blowing off less gas there will be even less tendency to blow off particles of faecal material lurking low down in the rectum. A more solid stool and a less gassy bowel habit represent the basis for the successful treatment of most pruritus ani (see Chapter 12 for instructions about how this can be achieved).

Keeping the perianal skin clean and dry also involves some simple daily routines. These are:

1. *Avoid washing the perianal skin with soap.* Water alone is sufficient. The detergent action of soap damages the skin's natural outer barrier and makes it even more susceptible to the negative effects of moisture and soiling. In addition, the perfumes and other chemicals that are used in soaps may cause a contact (allergic) dermatitis. Likewise, beware of 'baby wipes', which may also contain chemicals to which a hypersensitivity reaction can occur.

2. *Avoid powders and creams.* Powder, however sweet smelling, acts as a direct mechanical irritant to the perianal skin. Rather than drying up the moist areas, powder inevitably aggravates pruritus ani and should not be used.

Likewise, there is little reason to use creams and oint-ments on itchy skin. Ointments, in particular, are mois-turizing in nature and only make the skin soggy and prone to break down. What is more, preservatives and other chemicals in these creams and ointments may actually cause their own adverse reactions. In short, do not use any creams or ointments unless prescribed for you by a specialist.

3. *Dry the perianal skin gently but thoroughly* after a bowel action or shower. A soft towel or cloth is fine. However, when the perianal skin is broken and 'angry', even touching it can be unpleasant. In this situation dry-ing the perianal skin with a hairdryer (on cold!) is simple, soothing, and effective.

4. *Wear loose-fitting clothes wherever possible.* Even when this is impractical at work or when playing sport, try to get into loose-fitting clothing as soon as possible afterwards. Avoid underwear that contains man-made fibres; cotton is preferable. Even better, cotton boxer shorts allow the

maximum circulation of cooling air. Keeping the perianal skin cool is an important part of avoiding perspiration as a cause of pruritus ani.

What if things are out of control?

I have seen some raw, sore bottoms in my time! Long-standing soiling, itching, scratching, and weeping have left these tail ends red, ulcerated, and frankly unapproachable! Such individuals are understandably desperate.

Even though the basic rules of treatment still apply no matter how severe the situation, healing of this raw skin and relief from itching and burning pain may take days and weeks. In this situation I do recommend the use of a strong steroid cream—I use 0.1 per cent betamethasone cream—to heal the broken perianal skin and provide prompt relief.

A brief warning about steroid creams! Long-term use of steroid creams can cause permanent skin damage and encourages dependence, a kind of steroid 'addiction' where itching cannot be controlled by any other means. Steroid creams should never be used day in, day out for any considerable length of time. Rather, they should be used sparingly, a thin smear once or twice a day only for no more than one or two weeks. By this time, the basic steps of maintaining a solid stool, and keeping the skin clean and dry, etc. should be in place. The steroid cream can then be weaned off over another one to two weeks and used only occasionally in cases of emergency. Deterioration in the pruritus should prompt a serious review of the basic strategies and not just a return to using steroid creams!

Do haemorrhoids cause pruritus ani?

The answer is no and yes. Haemorrhoids cause bleeding, prolapse, and, when thrombosed, sudden pain. Rarely, however, are they the main cause of an itchy bottom! It is true that long-standing prolapse can be associated with some mucus discharge, which creates perianal moisture and can contribute to pruritus ani. Even in this situation the prominent complaints remain prolapse and bleeding, with the itching only a secondary issue. In other words, if itching is your main symptom, haemorrhoids—even if you have some—are unlikely to be the explanation.

Pruritus ani and anal fissure—a bad combination

Many people who suffer from chronic anal fissure (see Chapter 5) actively pursue a soft bowel motion so as to avoid the pain of passing something more solid. As a result, they frequently leave the toilet after emptying their bowels with a residue of soft faeces and then frequently experience post-defaecation soiling with pruritus. Many of these individuals, unaware that they have an underlying anal fissure, visit me complaining of the itching rather than the pain.

The basis of treating their pruritus is no different from any other person with common or garden variety pruritus ani. They need to pursue a more solid stool consistency in search of more complete rectal evacuation. Unfortunately, this may then cause pain and bleeding associated with their bowel action. In other words, if their motions are soft, they will have soiling and pruritus; if their motions are hard, they will have pain and bleeding!

The correct solution in this situation is to treat the anal fissure (as outlined in Chapter 5) and permit the individual to pursue a solid stool consistency. Where anal fissure and pruritus ani coexist, the only prospect for long-term anal comfort rests with correction of the anal fissure and the pursuit of solid stools.

Summary: Treating common or garden variety pruritus ani

1. Exclude or treat pinworm and fungal infections.
2. Pursue a solid stool consistency (see Chapter 12).
3. Keep the perianal skin clean and dry:
   (a) Bathe with water only (no soap).
   (b) Avoid creams and powders.
   (c) Dry gently but thoroughly after washing.
   (d) Wear loose-fitting clothing/natural fibres.
4. Sparing use only of strong steroid creams for severe flare-ups.

7
Bloating and irritable bowel syndrome

People—patients and doctors alike—are naturally drawn towards mechanical explanations for their symptoms. A blockage, a twist, a kink, adhesions, compression. We like to be able to visualize the cause of our complaints in these generally simple terms and imagine an equally simple, mechanical solution.

The concept of uncoordinated, excessive, or even deficient activity of the intestinal muscle tube is a whole lot harder to grasp. And the realization that there may not be a straightforward 'quick fix' tablet or operation can be just as hard to accept.

Yet this sort of muscular incoordination is precisely what causes so many abdominal and bowel symptoms. There is no narrowing to be seen on barium X-ray, no obstruction visible on colonoscopy, no mass or tumour on CT scan (a special form of X-ray), and no relief after adhesions have been divided surgically. The symptoms are certainly real: abdominal bloating and distension, crampy abdominal pains, episodes of diarrhoea or constipation (or both), nausea, and even vomiting. But the cause cannot be readily seen and all the explanations and reassurances in the world often fail to satisfy.

The gastrointestinal tract is a long, muscular tube that starts at the back of the throat and continues without interruption down to the external anal verge. The lining cells vary in appearance and function from gullet to stomach, from stomach to small intestine, from small to large intestine, and even from large intestine to anus. Some parts are narrow and some parts are wide but the intestinal muscle layer is present throughout. It is regularly called upon to propel food and other intestinal contents as well as to store faeces in a socially appropriate way! One way or another, the intestinal muscle tube is always at work either propelling or holding on to its contents and all the time reacting to changes in our diet, our medications, and our levels of exercise and stress.

It is hardly surprising—at least to me—that problems can arise from failure of this muscular tube to 'get it right'. Abnormal activity of the intestinal muscle tube is properly called 'gastrointestinal dysmotility'. A more common description is **irritable bowel syndrome**.

A diagnosis of irritable bowel syndrome is widely used and seems to mean different things to different doctors as well as to different patients. It is often applied to abdominal and bowel symptoms when no other cause is found and it is therefore prone to be overused. As a result, it has become a 'throw away' diagnosis for patients in the 'too hard' basket. Irritable bowel syndrome has become devalued as a legitimate diagnosis. Treatment, as well as all medical interest, seems to stop as soon as this label is attached.

Those of you with irritable bowel syndrome can attest to the fact that this is a distressing group of complaints. It is every bit as real as colitis and cancer, only much harder to diagnose with confidence. Importantly, it is nowhere near as serious or dangerous. It does, however, deserve more detailed understanding and a rational approach to treatment.

Are my symptoms due to irritable bowel syndrome?

One of the most difficult aspects of dealing with this condition is the myriad of ways in which it may present itself, all depending upon which parts of the gastrointestinal tract are most affected. You may recognize your own symptoms from one or more of the following descriptions of the common patterns of irritable bowel syndrome.

Gastroparesis

This describes predominant involvement of the stomach and very upper parts of the small intestine. Typically, there is upper abdominal bloating and nausea after meals due to distension of the stomach. This appears to be due to a failure of the stomach and duodenum to empty properly after a meal. Individuals affected by these symptoms often find certain foods—typically, these are fatty foods such as dairy products and fried foods—prone to provoke their complaints.

Other possible causes of these symptoms such as peptic ulcer or gallstones should be considered and excluded by means of gastroscopy (a telescopic view of the stomach achieved by swallowing a flexible, fibre-optic endoscope) and abdominal ultrasound scan. If gastroparesis is suspected, aggravating food should be avoided and stomach emptying assisted with the use of medications such as cisapride, domperidone, or metaclopramide.

Colonic inertia

An underactive colon causes constipation and abdominal bloating. This is described in detail in Chapter 4. There is considerable overlap between this variant of irritable bowel syndrome and so-called slow transit constipation, and treatment, in particular, is identical. It may be appropriate first to exclude more serious large intestinal conditions—polyps and cancer, in particular—by means of a barium X-ray or a colonoscopy examination.

Urgency and diarrhoea

In my own practice, this is the most common pattern of irritable bowel syndrome since it usually presents with incontinence. This is described in detail in Chapter 3 as the principal cause of urgency and incontinence of faeces.

This variant of irritable bowel syndrome is caused by episodic bursts of colonic muscle overactivity which occur as an excessive reaction to any of the usual stimuli that provoke colonic contraction in all of us (namely eating, exercising, and stress). Other causes of diarrhoea can be ruled out by testing the stool for infection or by looking for colitis at colonoscopy.

Treatment is aimed at achieving a firmer, slower-moving stool by changes in diet or by the introduction of anti-diarrhoeal medication (see Chapter 12). Irritable bowel syndrome causing urgency, diarrhoea, and incontinence generally responds very well to this simple strategy.

Alternating constipation and diarrhoea

Now this is a real challenge! These poor people don't know at the beginning of any day or week what lies ahead, at least from a bowel perspective. Will it be a burst of loose stool and a frantic rush to the nearest toilet? Or will it be a day (or more) of bloating and discomfort with little or no urge to have a bowel action? If they try to help the diarrhoea with medication they rapidly become constipated; if they take a laxative to get going again they might be humiliated by the urgent result.

Fortunately, this is not a common pattern as most people with irritable bowel syndrome suffer either predominant constipation or predominant diarrhoea. When the two occur in approximately equal proportions, treatment becomes particularly difficult.

Serious causes such as bowel cancer should be excluded by colonoscopy. The clue to successful treatment is the careful identification of aggravating influences in diet or lifestyle. Once these are identified, sufferers can generally begin to predict when problems might be brewing. More importantly, they come to realize that their bowel symptoms are just a reflection of their own individual response to changes in their environment and not a sign of a serious underlying disease. The irritable bowel syndrome doesn't go away but the sufferer can learn to accept it and learn to adjust.

Abdominal pain and distension

Uncoordinated spasms of the intestinal muscle tube can cause quite severe abdominal pain. The contracted or 'spastic' segment may, in effect, block the intestine at that point. As normal intestinal contractions continue down to the point of spasm and blockage, the intestine up-stream can become distended by gas and faeces. This pattern of irritable bowel syndrome is characterized by abdominal pain and bloating.

The pain may be quite localized and quite variable in its location depending on the point of spasm. The distended segment may also be uncomfortable or even frankly painful. This is usually felt in the right lower abdomen since the point of maximal distension is usually the caecum, the very first part of the large intestine.

Once again, this is a difficult pattern of irritable bowel syndrome to manage. If there is any suspicion of mechanical large intestinal obstruction, then a colonoscopy or barium X-ray will rule this out.

If there is an associated tendency towards constipation (in other words the pattern of colonic inertia) then laxative therapy is often helpful. If there is co-existent urgency and diarrhoea, then diet and anti-diarrhoeal therapies may be beneficial. Reassurance and the identification of any aggravating factors remain critical in helping sufferers of this pattern of irritable bowel syndrome adjust to their symptoms.

Stress and irritable bowel syndrome

None of us needs to be taught that stress can affect the way our intestines work! Who hasn't felt 'butterflies' in the stomach when nervous, or experienced abdominal cramps or even diarrhoea in anticipation of an important sporting or social event? Stress of all types affects our intestines. Marital problems, conflict in the workplace, financial worries, family matters, and even concerns about our own health act upon our bowel.

Often this produces urgency and diarrhoea but, equally, it may provoke bloating and constipation. One patient who I recall vividly, a woman in her fifties, suffered from severe slow transit constipation, not opening her bowels for over ten days without the use of laxatives. Yet a phone call from her elderly and estranged father living in another city was enough to give her urgent diarrhoea with incontinence!

The truth is that all of us feel stressed to some extent at different times. In some people this manifests as tension headaches; in others it might even be as depression. How our intestines respond to the stresses around us is all part of what makes us unique individuals. Often, it is those people who are striving to do many things, juggling stresses at home and at work, who fall victim to irritable bowel syndrome.

It is simply not practical to tell these 'high achievers' to wrap themselves in cotton wool or to learn to relax or take it easy. They won't and sometimes they can't!

The critical step in stress-induced irritable bowel syndrome is for the sufferers themselves to recognize the link between stresses in their environment and the workings of their intestine. Only rarely do these individuals take the time to reflect upon the myriad of decisions, deadlines, and dramas that fill their days! Once they do, they can nearly always pinpoint the added stress that has tipped their bowels into one pattern of irritable bowel syndrome or other.

Anxiety and worry are potent stresses in our lives. If we are anxious or worried about our health and, in this case, about why our bowels are playing up or about what might be causing abdominal pain and distension, irritable bowel syndrome only gets worse. Once we make that critical connection between our symptoms and the anxiety, nervousness, or even excitement that is causing them, problems start to ease off.

The realization that stress provokes symptoms is the first step towards breaking the self-perpetuating cycle of anxiety and irritable bowel syndrome. Confirmation that there is no serious underlying bowel disorder by performing some or all of the special tests already discussed comes second. Many times I have seen patients with long-standing irritable bowel syndrome in whom a whole barrage of expensive and undignified tests has been repeated every few years.

And the reason is that the connection between their stresses and anxieties and their actual symptoms has never been cemented. The negative tests reassure them for a short while only, but within a few years (add another child, add a larger mortgage, add a promotion to a more responsible position at work) the symptoms are just as bad or even worse, and all the old anxieties about what is causing them surface again.

Breaking this cycle of expensive investigation and temporary reassurance relies upon achieving a deeper appreciation of how every individual's intestinal function can be affected by the stresses and strains of ordinary living.

8
Diverticular disease of the colon

In the large intestine, a diverticulum is a kind of 'blow-out' of the intestinal wall. The thin inner lining of the wall bulges out through a tiny defect in the muscle layer creating what amounts to a 'bubble' on the outer surface of the colon. The individual diverticulum is a thin-walled sac or balloon that communicates with the main lumen of the colon.

Diverticular disease describes the occurrence of one or more diverticula of the large intestine. The rectum is never affected, only the colon. And within the colon, it is the sigmoid colon that is generally most severely involved. Hence we often hear this condition referred to as 'sigmoid diverticular disease'.

Diverticular disease is a common condition in Western countries (Australia, Canada, New Zealand, the United Kingdom, the USA, and Western Europe). It can appear in people in their thirties and forties but generally becomes progressively more common as we get older. In this sense, it may be a degenerative process, more and more diverticula 'blowing-out' as the colonic muscle ages and weakens.

There have been many theories as to why diverticular disease occurs but none has ever been conclusively established. The fact that this is common in Western countries, however, has been generally taken to mean that it has something to do with our Western—traditionally low fibre—diets.

On their own, the diverticula don't cause any symptoms. Many, many people with diverticular disease never

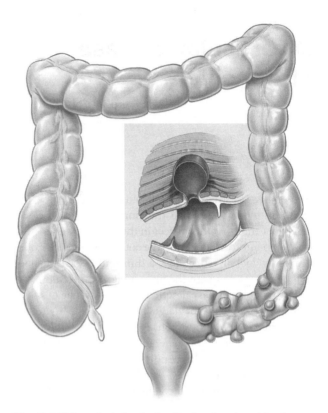

Fig. 8.1 Thin-walled diverticula affecting the sigmoid colon.

even know that they have it. Their condition may be found incidentally during a colonoscopy or a barium enema X-ray arranged for quite unrelated reasons. When diverticular disease does cause problems it can do so in a number of ways.

Diverticulitis

This term describes the situation where diverticular disease becomes complicated by inflammation and infection.

The thin-walled sacs can rupture (referred to as **perforation**), resulting in escape of bowel content—gas and faecal particles. Usually, the perforation is tiny, allowing escape of only minute amounts of gas or faeces. But even this sort of micro-perforation can be enough to cause intense inflammation around the offending diverticulum.

Since the usual point of perforation is in the mid- to lower sigmoid colon, the first complaint is often pain in the left lower abdomen. Irritation of the bowel by this infected and inflamed process now gathering outside the sigmoid colon can result in a degree of diarrhoea. But the main symptom is abdominal pain, usually worst in the left lower abdomen.

When individuals with diverticulitis are examined by their doctor, they are often found to have a fever and clear-cut abdominal tenderness over the area of perforation. The correct treatment for this mild to moderate attack of diverticulitis is a course of antibiotics. These generally settle the infection and inflammation without the need for any further treatment. Only if such episodes were to become progressively more frequent and disruptive would a more radical approach, such as surgical removal of the diverticular segment, be considered. Luckily, most people who suffer from diverticulitis fit into the mild to moderate category and go through life never needing more than an occasional course of antibiotics.

Severe diverticulitis and abscesses

Needless to say, not all episodes of diverticulitis are only of mild to moderate severity. When the degree of perforation is greater, there is more extensive escape of bowel content and there may be quite severe local inflammation and even abscess formation. An abscess in an obvious collection of pus, in this case situated alongside the colon at the point of diverticular perforation. In this event pain is understandably more severe, the fever even higher, and abdominal tenderness more pronounced. The severely inflamed segment of colon—with or without an abscess—may even produce a lump or mass that can be felt when examining the abdomen.

Severe diverticulitis and abscesses represent a serious situation and prompt control of the infection is necessary if even more extensive and generalized infection is to be avoided. This sort of episode generally requires admission to hospital and the use of intravenous antibiotics (administered through an intravenous drip).

A CT scan of the abdomen might identify an obvious abscess around the bowel. Using modern techniques, expert radiologists can often insert drains into such an abscess under local anaesthetic.

The combination of intravenous antibiotics and radiological drainage of any abscess, when present, may bring a severe episode under control, avoiding the need for an emergency operation. Just the same, a severe episode such as this represents a clear warning to both patient and surgeon: Don't wait for another attack! After even just one major attack of diverticulitis, the writing is generally on the wall! Get the diverticular disease removed as soon as the infection has fully settled!

Generalized peritonitis

This is the extreme end of diverticulitis. Rarely, a major escape of bowel content may occur when a diverticulum perforates. More often, an abscess that has formed around a perforated diverticulum gets so large that is ruptures, spreading pus and infection around the abdominal cavity. This is accompanied by a sudden increase in the severity and the extent of pain and by a dramatic increase in the severity and extent of abdominal tenderness. We call this **generalized peritonitis** and it represents a dire surgical emergency.

An operation is required immediately, before intra-abdominal infection provokes an even more widespread total body response. Once this total body response starts, it cannot be readily reversed, even with appropriate surgery to control the peritonitis. When an operation is undertaken too late, it is a bit like removing a faulty electrical appliance after the house has already been set on fire! The initial cause may have been corrected but the 'fire' still rages on.

In the event of such an emergency an operation usually involves removing the diseased diverticular segment and washing out as much of the contamination as possible with warm, sterile water. Some surgeons will attempt to rejoin the bowel but many prefer a more cautious approach, closing over the lower part (the rectum) and bringing the upper part out through the abdominal wall as a colostomy (or 'bag'). Only when the infection has fully settled and the patient has recovered completely—often more than three or four months later—can the bowel be rejoined in yet another operation.

Because emergency operations for diverticulitis might involve the construction of a colostomy and because the subsequent operation to rejoin the bowel is also a very major undertaking, it makes good sense to prevent an emergency situation from ever developing in the first place. If you have had repeated attacks of diverticulitis or even just one that was severe, you might be well advised to consider a preventative operation to remove the diverticular segment and rejoin the bowel in a planned manner. This will reduce the risk of you needing a colostomy as well as the risk of you needing a second operation. The advice of a surgeon experienced in the treatment of diverticulitis is essential.

Diverticular stricture

Repeated episodes of diverticulitis can, over time, lead to fibrous narrowing of the sigmoid colon. This is often only detected when the individual undergoes a colonoscopy or barium enema X-ray and the narrowed point becomes obvious. Only occasionally, the diverticular stricture can cause the symptoms of colonic obstruction—crampy lower abdominal pain (colic) and abdominal bloating.

Even though a diverticular stricture is benign, the presence of any narrowing in the colon always raises the possibility of a cancer being present. If the colonoscope cannot be passed through the stricture to examine the entire surface of the colon properly, it may not be possible to exclude completely a colorectal cancer. Even if this can be achieved, regular surveillance is necessary resulting in the need for repeated colonoscopies and/or barium enema X-rays.

As a result, many patients with tight diverticular strictures require or prefer planned resection of their diverticular disease. Interestingly, once people have recovered from resection of their stricture, they often comment on how much better is their bowel habit and how much more comfortable they are in general.

Haemorrhage

Dramatic, fresh bleeding from the colon is uncommon but it is a well-recognized phenomenon. And diverticular disease is one of the most common causes of such colonic haemorrhage. Infection along the neck of the diverticulum may erode into a critically placed blood vessel causing fresh bleeding back into the colon.

Luckily, haemorrhage from diverticular disease generally subsides of its own accord and may never recur. But if such bleeding fails to stop or if repeated bouts of haemorrhage continue to occur, resection of the offending segment of colon becomes a life-saving operation.

Of course, it can be difficult to know exactly which diverticulum is responsible for the bleeding even after extensive testing! As a result, surgeons are likely to remove a somewhat longer segment of colon than they might otherwise have done, to be as sure as they can that they have removed the bleeding point.

It is important to emphasize that haemorrhage from diverticular disease is not common and that, even when it does occur, it generally subsides of its own accord. Surgery for uncontrolled or repeated episodes of bleeding from diverticular disease is rarely necessary.

Diet and diverticular disease

Because diverticular disease is such a common problem in the Western world yet not so in the developing world, diet and, in particular, dietary fibre have been implicated in its cause and treatment. Proponents of diet therapy for diverticular disease believe that complications such as diverticulitis and bleeding can be prevented by strict adherence to a special diet.

But the answer is not a simple high fibre diet. In fact, certain sources of dietary fibre might even aggravate diverticular disease and provoke complications!

The current recommendation for individuals who have had symptoms from their diverticular disease is that they should pursue a diet with soluble fibre (soft, non-irritant) and strictly avoid insoluble fibre (roughage). A dietician can provide a detailed list of food types that belong to these different categories of fibre.

What is the evidence that diet makes a difference in diverticular disease? Not too good, I'm afraid! As with all dietary recommendations, those that we give for diverticular disease also need to be 'taken with a pinch of salt'!

Diet is clearly only one element in the complex puzzle of diverticular disease. The thought of my patients painstakingly sifting through each meal, peeling tomatoes, de-pipping grapes, avoiding certain foods altogether, and generally missing out on the full enjoyment of their meals—with no guarantee whatsoever that all this will prevent episodes of diverticulitis—fills me with horror. Just as bad is the image of other people, without any symptoms of diverticular disease, restricting their diet on the advice of well-meaning doctors, dieticians, and friends. This is plainly ridiculous.

In the quest for preventative strategies and, in particular, strategies free from the use of drugs and medications, many people are turned into dietary cripples. They become unable to eat even a single meal without detailed inspection, meticulous dissection, and high anxiety that, despite their best efforts, they've done the wrong thing!

Diet does have a part to play in the treatment of diverticular disease. But this part should never be allowed to interfere with the basic notion that food is meant to be eaten and enjoyed!

Diverticular disease or irritable bowel syndrome?

As I said at the beginning of Chapter 7 on irritable bowel syndrome, it is a basic element of human nature to attribute our symptoms to some visible, mechanical abnormality. As a result, the presence of diverticula, whether seen on colonoscopy or on barium enema X-ray, is often regarded as the explanation of troublesome abdominal and gastrointestinal symptoms just because they are clearly visible and easily explained. Both diverticular disease and irritable bowel syndrome are common and, not suprisingly, many people who have one will also have the other. But which one is causing the symptoms?

Put simply, a pattern of troublesome diarrhoea and short-lived episodes of abdominal pain points towards irritable bowel syndrome. A pattern of more prolonged bouts of pain, lasting days rather than hours, accompanied by fever and persisting abdominal tenderness, which requires antibiotics, points towards diverticulitis.

This distinction is important. I've seen many people referred to me for consideration of a bowel resection whose long-standing abdominal pain and loose stools have been attributed to their diverticular disease and who have been treated over many years with a high fibre diet and repeated courses of antibiotics. Yet the main cause of their symptoms has always been their irritable bowel and a change of treatment towards a reduction in dietary fibre and the use of simple anti-diarrhoeal medication has dramatically improved their situation.

As I have pointed out already, it is unwise to allow diverticular disease to progress to the point of a major perforation. Repeated bouts should be taken as a warning that a more serious attack may soon follow. Just the same, removing a segment of diverticular disease is unlikely to correct an irritable bowel! And this is a major operation to go through, only to find out afterwards that the symptoms have not gone away.

Assessment of your symptoms by doctors experienced in the treatment of intestinal diseases should help prevent unnecessary surgery if irritable bowel syndrome is your main problem. Equally, their opinion and advice should prevent unnecessary delays in recommending surgery for those of you with significant diverticular disease.

9
Dangerous creatures: Cancer, Crohn's disease, and ulcerative colitis

Like every other part of the human body, our gastrointestinal tract can fall victim to serious and life-threatening diseases. In their early stages, many of these diseases produce symptoms that are not unlike those caused by the common anorectal conditions or irritable bowel syndrome as already discussed.

The following accounts of some well-known 'dangerous creatures' are, inevitably, only brief. They attempt to explain the causes of these conditions, alert you to their early symptoms, and encourage a sensible approach to whether or not to have further investigations. They also discuss, in simple terms, the treatments available. More detailed information can be obtained from your family doctor or from such organizations as your local cancer foundation or Crohn's and colitis association.

Cancer of the colon and rectum (colorectal cancer)

Cancers of the large intestine (colon and rectum) are a major cause of disability and death, especially in the Western world, where more people die each year from colorectal cancer than from either breast cancer or prostate cancer. In Australia alone, more than 10,000 new cases of colorectal cancer are diagnosed each year and there are, annually, over 4500 deaths from this condition. Undeniably, this is a major health problem for the Western world.

What is colorectal cancer?

A cancer is an abnormal overgrowth of one type or other of the body's cells. Cancers can arise in the cells of the skin, in the cells of the breast tissue, the prostate gland, the airways of the lung, the lymphatic cells, etc. Colorectal cancer arises in the cells that line the inner surface of the large intestine (colon and rectum).

What makes all cancers so dangerous is the fact that they continue to grow unchecked. They may become large, they may erode into surrounding tissue, and, finally, they may spread through blood vessels and lymph channels to other parts of the body. Wherever they settle and survive—by overwhelming the body's local resistance forces—they also grow unchecked.

The cancer itself and any of its deposits use up a disproportionate amount of the body's energy supply, growing at the expense of other parts of the body not yet affected or involved by the cancer. Gradually, the individual affected by widespread cancer becomes weakened and wasted as the cancer cells consume energy and nutrients.

In colorectal cancer the growth or primary tumour starts on the inner lining of the intestine and grows locally. It protrudes internally into the intestinal lumen and invades deeply through the muscle wall of the intestine. It may erode through the full thickness of the intestinal wall and attach itself to nearby structures such as other loops of small intestine, the bladder, or the vagina in women.

Spread from colorectal cancer—called secondary deposits, secondaries, or metastases—usually travels first to the nearby lymph nodes, also referred to as lymph glands. Beyond this, cancer may spread to the liver and in some cases to lung, bone, and elsewhere.

How do you get colorectal cancer?

Colorectal cancer starts in the cells that line the inner surface of the large intestine. Normally, these cells multiply, die, and disappear in a furious but orderly fashion.

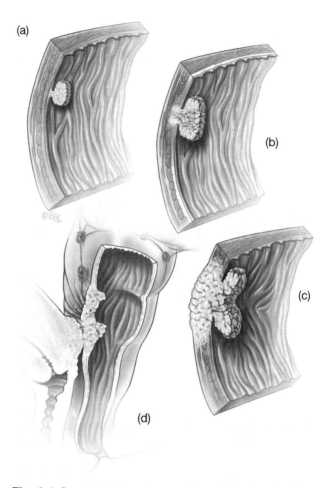

Fig. 9.1 Growth of a bowel cancer through the bowel wall, showing progression from polyp (a) to invasive cancer (b), and increasing depth of invasion by cancer (c and d).

Each cell splits into two identical 'daughter' cells that carry on the usual work of the colon, absorbing a little water to dry out the faeces and secreting a little mucus to act as a lubricating agent. There are many millions of cells lining the large intestine, all multiplying, dying, and disappearing every moment of the day.

It is not at all surprising that, with all this multiplication and cell division going on, some cells get it wrong. In other words, a faulty attempt at multiplication can easily produce two daughter cells that are not quite like the parent and might not behave in quite such an orderly fashion. Major problems in cell multiplication usually result in cells that are so abnormal that they simply cannot survive. These daughter cells are doomed from the start, and die off and disappear. More subtle problems in cell multiplication are not immediately fatal and these daughter cells can survive and start multiplying in their own right to produce equally abnormal daughter cells of their own.

Luckily, every cell in the body is equipped to deal with precisely such mistakes in cell multiplication. The cells have special systems in place for the early detection of errors in cell multiplication and for correcting them so that the resulting daughter cells end up looking just like 'mum'.

Sometimes, however, the sheer number of multiplication errors overwhelms these defence mechanisms. Alternatively, the defence mechanisms themselves might be inherently weak or absent. In these circumstances, the faulty cell multiplication goes unchecked, the abnormal daughter cells survive and multiply, and the pathway leading to colorectal cancer has begun.

The initial, visible abnormality in colorectal cancer is not a fully formed cancer at all but a small nodule or **polyp**. In fact, at this early stage, the polyp is usually benign, in other words incapable of invading the bowel wall or spreading more widely. These polyps are called adenomas; they are not yet cancerous. But within them, their abnormal cells are also furiously multiplying, and it only takes one or two additional errors of cell multiplication to escape detection and correction for the growth of that polyp to lose all restraint. This sequence of undetected errors of cell division, from normal to benign polyp to cancer, explains almost all of the colorectal cancer we see.

Who gets colorectal cancer?

Colorectal cancer is much more common in the Western world (Australia, Canada, New Zealand, the United Kingdom, the USA, and Western Europe) than it is in Asia and Africa. It is hard to escape the conclusion that something about our Western lifestyle has a part to play! In fact, there is now plenty of evidence to suggest that a diet rich in fat and lacking in fruit and vegetables contributes to this high rate of colorectal cancer in Western countries. It is probable that the chemical environment inside the large bowel that results from this high fat, low fibre diet favours faulty cell multiplication, overwhelming the otherwise normal early-detection-and-correction systems in place. This may also explain why smokers appear to have an increased likelihood of developing colorectal cancer—swallowed smoke might adversely affect the chemical environment inside the large intestine.

Yet we all too frequently see colorectal cancer in people leading thoroughly healthy lifestyles—high fibre diet, non-smoker, regular exercise! Surely their colorectal cancer can't also be attributed to bad Western habits? And, sadly, we also see colorectal cancer in young people, in their thirties and forties (or younger) who haven't yet had enough exposure to these so-called risk factors to cause their cancers. What explains the development of colorectal cancer in the young and the health conscious?

Unfortunately, we don't yet fully understand why these people, in particular, get colorectal cancer. Only a small number—perhaps 5 per cent or 1 in 20—of all cases of colorectal cancer appear to belong to families with an inherited predisposition to colorectal cancer. In these families there is a genetic abnormality—an inbuilt weakness of the detection-and-correction system—that leaves affected individuals almost certain to develop colorectal cancer at some stage of their lives. And these individuals then have the potential to pass on this genetic abnormality and the associated risk of colorectal cancer to

1 in 2 of their children. This may result in generation after generation of people in the one family who have developed colorectal cancer and undergone surgery.

Even if you do not have a strong family history of colorectal cancer (perhaps only your mother or father, or a solitary brother or sister), you may still carry an increased risk of developing the disease. This risk appears to be higher if more than one relative has been affected and if the relatives who have been affected developed their colorectal cancer at young ages.

If you do have a family history of colorectal cancer, as well as, say, breast or uterine (endometrial) cancer, you should consult your family doctor to ascertain both your risk of belonging to an inherited colorectal cancer family and your overall risk of developing the disease. Your doctor can then advise you on what tests should be done to detect colorectal cancer at the earliest possible stage and whether or not more complex, genetic testing for a hereditary sydrome is appropriate. You may also be able to obtain helpful information from an inherited colorectal cancer registry or familial polyposis registry in your own area.

Despite all this talk of inheriting colorectal cancer, at least three-quarters of all cases do not even have a family history of this disease to suggest why they were prone to develop it in the first place! A few may have been predisposed to it by virtue of having ulcerative colitis or Crohn's disease (see later in this chapter). But we are still left with the fact that we do not yet know why most people with colorectal cancer actually get it. And since we don't know why, we really don't know who is going to get it until they turn up in our surgeries and clinics with the symptoms of this dangerous disease.

What are the symptoms of colorectal cancer?

If we could only detect colorectal cancer earlier on in its course there is no doubt that we would be able to cure more of those people who develop it. It is true that in some people, the cancer is already widespread when the first complaints and symptoms appear. Equally, it is true that colorectal cancer can produce all sorts of different symptoms that might not at first suggest where the problem is lurking.

Yet, time and time again, doctors are confronted with people who for many months have been experiencing the characteristic symptoms of a colorectal cancer without seeking medical advice. Embarrassment, a busy schedule, and even anxiety that the cause might be serious can keep them away until symptoms can no longer be ignored. And by then, it may truly be too late!

So what are the symptoms you should be looking for? Put simply, they are rectal bleeding and anaemia, an altered bowel habit, and abdominal bloating.

The surface of a colorectal cancer is easily traumatized and can readily *bleed*. For the blood to be visible either on the surface of a bowel action or, more often, mixed in with it, the cancer really has to be situated relatively close to the anus. Cancers in the rectum and sigmoid colon (and occasionally in the descending colon) may produce visible blood in the bowel motion. This is quite different from the very fresh blood seen on toilet paper or dripping into the toilet bowl that results from haemorrhoids or anal fissure.

Cancers that are situated in the caecum, and ascending and transverse colons can still bleed but, by the time the blood reaches the outside world, it has been altered and darkened, and is generally disguised within the bowel motion. The only external sign might be a dark or, occasionally, black colour to the stool.

But steady blood loss from colorectal cancers can deplete the blood of its red cells and the oxygen-carrying haemoglobin. This results in *anaemia*. The affected individuals look pale and may be lethargic, easily tired, and breathless on light exertion. Although many different conditions can be responsible for causing anaemia, colorectal cancer is a common and clearly important one. Your doctor will know only too well the significance of anaemia, its various causes, and how to investigate it thoroughly.

As the colorectal cancer grows into the bowel lumen and invades then encircles the bowel wall, it causes a definite narrowing. This blocks the free passage of content through this area, resulting in loss of the bowel's regular pattern of contraction and action. There can be a sense of *constipation and abdominal bloating* as the colon upstream from the cancer distends with gas and stool. Laxatives may be used to get things going resulting in a powerful, loose bowel action as the build-up of stool is forced through the narrowed segment. This results in pattern of *alternating constipation and diarrhoea.*

These symptoms are more likely to occur if the colorectal cancer affects the relatively narrow sigmoid, descending, and transverse areas of the colon. Cancers in the large, capacious regions of the large intestine (caecum and rectum) tend to be a little different.

In the caecum, the tumour may grow slowly without causing symptoms and blockage. Equally, cancers close to the entry point of the small intestine—the ileo-caecal junction—can produce symptoms of small intestinal obstruction such as crampy abdominal pains shortly after meals accompanied by noisy gurgling and even tinkling sounds coming from the abdomen. The combination of these symptoms of intestinal blockage and anaemia strongly suggest a cancer affecting the caecum.

In the rectum, a cancer may produce a constant sensation of the need to have a bowel action. The rectum is very sensitive to the presence of material within it; when the 'material' is a cancer and that cancer is firmly attached to the rectal wall, no amount of pushing and straining will give relief. This sensation of incomplete evacuation—particularly when it is associated with rectal bleeding—should alert you to the possibility of an underlying rectal cancer.

Making the diagnosis

Once you see your doctor a number of procedures and investigations are likely to take place in an attempt to exclude or to confirm the possibility of a colorectal cancer as the cause of your symptoms. Your doctor will perform an internal rectal examination, an unpleasant but utterly vital first step. This will immediately detect any cancer low down in the rectum, greatly speeding up the process of further investigation and treatment.

Your doctor may also perform a rigid sigmoidoscopy, an internal inspection with a hollow, plastic telescope inserted about 15–20 cm (about 6–8 inches) into the rectum. This enables the rectum and sometimes the lower sigmoid colon to be seen and any abnormalities to be biopsied (a small sample is taken for examination by a pathologist).

More complete evacuation of the large intestine may be achieved by means of a colonoscopy, which is a long, flexible telescope that can be passed from the anus all the way around and even into the terminal ileum. The entire internal surface of the colon and rectum can be carefully inspected and any suspicious areas biopsied for confirmation.

The bowel has to be thoroughly cleaned—usually with the aid of strong laxatives of the osmotic (salty solution) variety—so that the bowel lining can be clearly seen. Most people find the process of bowel cleansing the most unsavoury part of the entire exercise! The passage of the colonoscope through the bowel is performed with the aid of sedation or even a general anaesthetic but few people recall it as an unpleasant experience.

An alternative to colonoscopy is a barium enema X-ray. Again, the bowel must be thoroughly cleaned before this X-ray, which involves inflation of the bowel by air and barium—a white, pasty substance which shows up clearly on the X-ray—through a tube passed into the lower rectum. During the X-ray, you are moved about upon a special X-ray table to tilt you head up, head down, or left or right side up. Sedation or anaesthesia is not usually required but the procedure is often uncomfortable. More importantly, it isn't, overall, quite as accurate as colonoscopy in the search for colorectal cancer and it is generally used only when colonoscopy has been incomplete or is simply unavailable.

What about scans? Ultrasound, CT, MRI! All of these scans can be used to assess the extent of spread of colorectal cancer. They can be used to assess how big is the primary cancer and how deeply invasive it is through the bowel wall. They are probably better, however, for determining the presence of more widespread involvement of the lymph nodes, liver, and lungs. Your doctor may well arrange these scans to be performed to exclude the possibility of widespread disease rather than because of any real suspicion that spread has already occurred. Such scans are now commonplace in the assessment of people with a newly diagnosed colorectal cancer.

Treating colorectal cancer

The term cancer strikes fear in the hearts of all who come in close contact with it. We know that cancers can kill but in the minds of some people, the diagnosis of colorectal cancer immediately spells certain death. This is not true; the majority of people newly diagnosed with colorectal cancer are, ultimately, cured.

But the treatment of colorectal cancer frequently requires major surgery, is often drawn out by chemotherapy and radiotherapy, and occasionally involves significant and permanent changes in lifestyle. And, as we know, it does not always succeed in achieving a cure.

The full range of treatment options, and all the various risks and benefits associated with them, is beyond the scope of this book. I will, however, attempt to cover the basic principles of treatment and summarize the main treatment methods. If you have been diagnosed with colorectal cancer, your doctors—family doctor, surgeon, oncologist, etc.—will be in the best position to advise you of the best treatment in your own, highly individual, situation.

In fact, this is a good way to start discussing the basic principles of treatment.

1. Every individual case requires its own individual treatment plan. No two cases of colorectal cancer will ever be exactly the same. As a group, we doctors depend heavily upon recognizing an individual situation and relating it to our personal and collective experience in similar situations. We know how people *usually* get on when they have this or that combination of clinical features. We deal with percentages and probabilities and frequently use them in recommending one treatment or another.

This might make us feel as if we are providing good, scientific advice but it can be very confusing for our patients: 'You told me that 50 per cent of people respond to this treatment, but are you advising me to have it or not?' Knowing what the treatment options are doesn't always help you know which one to choose!

The same is true for your doctors! There are always a multitude of factors that need to be weighed up in planning treatment: Where is the cancer? How advanced do we think it is? Does it appear to be growing rapidly or slowly? How fit for aggressive treatment is this patient? Where would it be best for him or her to have the treatment?

Your case is unique and you need to take part in the decision-making along with your doctors, family, and friends. Practical, useful information and clear communication are the keys to building mutual trust between you and your doctors. From this standpoint, treatment—however difficult—can generally be approached calmly and with confidence.

2. Surgical removal of the primary cancer with a safe margin of normal intestine around it remains the single most important step in treating colorectal cancer. Whatever other treatments you may undergo, the simple concept of cure by cutting it out still holds true. But surgery for colorectal cancer means major surgery—in all but a tiny number of the smallest of low rectal cancers, where it is sometimes possible to remove the cancer completely by operating entirely 'from below', in other words through the anus.

So curing colorectal cancer generally means major abdominal surgery. This often means a large incision, a potentially painful post-operative recovery, and a lengthy period of recuperation—up to six weeks to get back to 'normal'. Where the tumour is removed and the ends of the intestine are rejoined there may be a change in your bowel habit due to the length of intestine removed. There is also the risk of leakage from the new junction— fortunately infrequent—causing serious infection and requiring immediate re-operation.

When your surgeon is concerned that the new junction is at greater than usual risk of leakage, a temporary 'bag' (colostomy or ileostomy) may be constructed. Even though this is only temporary, it takes quite some getting used to and requires a second, fortunately much smaller, operation to close it which will allow your bowels to work in the usual manner again.

When colorectal cancer affects the lowest portion of the rectum, close to the anal sphincter muscles, it may not be possible to remove the cancer along with a safe margin around it and still rejoin the ends of the intestine. In this situation—now relatively rare in the era of advanced surgical techniques—curing colorectal cancer means *not* rejoining the intestine. In other words, this involves the construction of a permanent bag, or **stoma**.

A stoma may be a colostomy when the colon (large intestine) is used or an ileostomy when the ileum (small intestine) is used. It is an opening from the intestine to the skin of the abdomen. Intestinal contractions continue as usual but there is no rectum to store faeces and no sphincter muscles to keep the faeces inside. As a result, faeces pass directly through this stoma according to the pattern of your intestinal contractions. The faeces need to be collected in a plastic bag—or **pouch**—fastened to the skin around the stoma with an adhesive material. When the pouch is full it can be emptied, cleaned, and reattached; or can be thrown away and replaced completely, depending upon the type of pouch you are using.

It goes without saying that life with a stoma—temporary or permanent—requires major readjustment. Many issues need to be addressed: practical handling issues, dietary changes, altered body image, and self-esteem. Nurses expert in all these areas are called **enterostomal therapists**. They are as important as your surgeon in the post-operative recovery after stoma construction. No doubt your surgeon will direct you to an enterostomal therapist with whom he or she works very closely even before your surgery takes place.

The prospect of a permanent stoma is a frightening one for individuals newly diagnosed with colorectal cancer. Yet only lower rectal tumours are ever likely to require one on a permanent basis. It is a constant source of inspiration to me and a tribute to people's resolve and ability to adapt that virtually everyone who requires a permanent stoma manages with so little fuss and complaint.

It certainly isn't their 'first choice' but they get on with their lives almost as if nothing has happened. One patient of mine, a slim aerobics instructor in her early forties who had returned to work with her stoma, summed up her situation simply and with a smile: 'The bag is a drag!'

The full details of your surgery—all the risks, benefits, alternatives, and goals—need to be discussed in great detail before surgery. Your surgeon is in the best position to answer all these questions.

3. The word chemotherapy conjures up images of waif-like children, pale and bald, in the throes of aggressive treatment of leukaemia. Certainly, the chemotherapy used for some cancers can have these effects. But the drugs that have been found to be effective in colorectal cancer do not appear to be quite so toxic at standard doses. Mouth ulceration and diarrhoea appear to be the most common side-effects. Your oncologist will be able to give you a more detailed list of the potential side-effects of your chemotherapy. But which patients with colorectal cancer actually need chemotherapy? There are two basic scenarios in which chemotherapy may be used.

(a) *In support of surgery as part of treatment aimed at cure.* We call this **adjuvant** chemotherapy. It usually starts about four to six weeks after surgery and continues for about six months; it is used in individuals whose tumours have spread to lymph nodes. This can only be determined once the segment of intestine removed at surgery has been analysed by a pathologist. We know that those with spread to lymph nodes, in particular, are more likely to develop widespread colorectal cancer in the future than those whose cancer has not. Presumably, there must have been cancer cells within the blood-stream or the lymphatic vessels at the time of surgery which then went on to lodge in the liver, lungs, and bones but only appeared months or years down the track.

The idea of adjuvant chemotherapy is to kill these cells floating about in the circulation before they lodge in other organs or while they are still only very tiny deposits of tumour in these organs.

Scientific evidence suggests that the use of adjuvant chemotherapy after surgery increases the likelihood of cure for patients with colorectal cancer that has spread to lymph nodes by only about 20–30 per cent. Not a great added success rate but worthwhile in those young enough and fit enough to withstand the side-effects of chemotherapy. Again, your surgeon and your oncologist will be able to guide you in this matter.

(b) *In the treatment of widespread colorectal cancer.* We call this **palliative** chemotherapy. This is not designed to cure, only to control unpleasant symptoms and to prolong and enhance quality of life. Many people—especially older people or those who have had a bad experience witnessing chemotherapy being given to dying friends or relatives—decide against chemotherapy in this situation. Others press on with more aggressive treatment, hoping for extra months of life to spend and enjoy with their family and friends. Like all other aspects of the treatment of colorectal cancer, the decision to use palliative chemotherapy is a highly individual one.

4. Like chemotherapy, radiotherapy can be used in both adjuvant (curative) and palliative (non-curative) situations. But it is almost exclusively used in rectal cancer and almost never in colonic cancer.

One of the major problems facing patients with rectal cancer—and their surgeons—is the risk of local recurrence of cancer. This describes the situation where cancer reappears not at a distance—such as in the liver or lung—but in the pelvis itself, attached to the muscles and bones alongside where the rectal cancer was before it was surgically removed. Even though the surgeon thought that all the cancer had been removed, cancer cells in the vicinity can obviously survive and thrive, and reappear months or years later. Local recurrence of rectal cancer is almost impossible to eradicate even by radical re-operative surgery. And even radiotherapy in this setting can only be considered palliative, that is, not for cure.

What makes radiotherapy in rectal cancer treatment exciting is its use as an adjuvant agent, that is, in support of surgery for a cure. These days it is most often given before surgery, shrinking the primary cancer and, hopefully, destroying those other cancer cells in the nearby vicinity that surgery alone cannot remove. Strong evidence now supports the use of radiotherapy in combination with surgery for large rectal cancers or those very low in the rectum. In these cases, this combination reduces local recurrence of cancer and makes long-term cure more likely than with surgery alone.

What if my cancer is not curable?

Unfortunately, there are some people whose colorectal cancer is clearly beyond cure. This situation may be apparent even at the time of first diagnosis although it more commonly develops in the course of follow-up after a previous treatment for the primary cancer. Where there has been extensive spread to the liver or lung, or where there are widespread nodules of cancer within the abdomen, colorectal cancer can no longer reasonably be cured.

In these situations, heroic surgery is rarely appropriate although smaller operations and other treatments such as chemotherapy and radiotherapy may still be useful for symptom control. The emphasis must be on achieving good palliation, focusing on quality of life and respect for the dignity of the patient. Wonderful support services now exist for the care of terminally ill patients, enabling nursing care and control of symptoms with minimal disruption to normal routine. Your family doctor will know of the most appropriate palliative care services in your locality.

Preventing colorectal cancer

We know that the earlier in the course of the cancer that we can start treatment, the more likely we are to be able to cure it. Unfortunately, by the time most colorectal cancer starts to cause symptoms—bleeding, anaemia, altered bowel habit, bloating, etc.—it has often already been present and growing for quite a long time. As a result, it may have already grown through the full thickness of the intestinal wall, have spread to lymph nodes, and might even have spread to liver, lung, and beyond.

If we are going to make any impact at all on the alarming number of deaths caused by colorectal cancer, it will not be because large numbers of people suddenly start turning up with symptoms three to six months earlier than at present! Of course, you must report the key symptoms early and you must not wait! But to reduce the number of deaths from colorectal cancer significantly, we have to start finding these cancers much, much earlier, before they start producing symptoms, even before the polyp has turned into a cancer!

And it *is* possible to do this! The ideal test is a colonoscopy—already described in this chapter. This test enables the entire lining of the colon and rectum to be seen, any small polyps to be removed, and larger polyps or even early cancers to be biopsied for confirmation. A benign polyp removed in this way is, in fact, a cancer of the future prevented!

Of course, the preparation, in particular, for this test can be an unpleasant experience and colonoscopy is not without some risk. What is more, it isn't always readily available—there are many more people already waiting for their colonoscopy to be performed than there is available time to do them all!

But this is without doubt the best test currently available. Certainly, for those of you with an increased risk of colorectal cancer because of a previously diagnosed polyp or colorectal cancer, or because of a known family history of colorectal cancer, *only a colonoscopy will do!* Ideally, you need to start tests at an early age—no later than 40 years old, in my opinion—and continue them regularly throughout life. Even if each test is totally normal, you should continue with a colonoscopy every five years.

What about those of us with no family history of colorectal cancer and no obvious increased risk of developing it? We are all said to be at 'average risk', yet over 70 per cent of all newly diagnosed cases of colorectal cancer are in people precisely like us, at average risk. We are the main body of colorectal cancer—and we want to know how to prevent it!

Even though colonoscopy is the best test, if we all start turning up at the age of 40 years expecting a colonoscopy to be performed and then repeated every five years, the medical system will be rapidly overwhelmed. Even worse, we would delay some people who already have symptoms of colorectal cancer from getting their colonoscopy done and will hold back the start of their all-important treatment.

One of two solutions, although neither is perfect, is to try to select people for colonoscopy on the basis of another, much more easily available, test. Such a test is available. We can test our own faeces for blood using a cheap and simple kit that can be used in the privacy of our own homes. If this test—the Faecal Occult Blood Test or **FOBT**—is positive for blood, there is an increased chance that we have a polyp or a colorectal cancer and colonoscopy should be performed. Obviously, if the FOBT is negative, colonoscopy should not be performed. It is generally recommended that the FOBT be repeated every year in people over the age of 40.

Often the colonoscopy is all-clear even though the FOBT was positive (false positive test). And, sadly, even when polyps and colorectal cancers are present, the FOBT can still be negative (false negative test). These inaccuracies can lead to unnecessary anxiety or misplaced relief and they make the FOBT a difficult test to recommend.

The other solution is to use a colonoscopy but not to use it as frequently as for those who are obviously at increased risk of colorectal cancer. Some advise that it be performed twice: at 50 years of age and again at 60 years; others advise that it only be used 'once in a lifetime'. If all of us who are only at average risk of developing colorectal cancer were to have just one colonoscopy at the age of 58 to 60 years, there would be a substantial drop in the number of cases of colorectal cancer and a substantial increase in the percentage of cases diagnosed early rather than late. Lives would be saved, operations avoided, colostomies prevented.

This, too, is an expensive exercise when spread out across the entire population. Currently, even the relatively wealthy Western countries appear to lack the resolve to commit the necessary resources to such a strategy aimed at preventing colorectal cancer. I believe that, in time, the reduction in surgery, chemotherapy and radiotherapy as well as the reduction in both hospitalisation and sheer time away from the workforce would more than compensate for the cost of prevention.

I can assure you that when I turn 50, I'll be arranging to have a colonoscopy and, even if it is normal, I will have it repeated at 60. I am convinced that colonoscopy represents the best available strategy for preventing this serious and dangerous disease. And, having witnessed the distress and suffering colorectal cancer causes, I am convinced that the costs involved in preventing it are well justified.

I cannot emphasize enough the importance of being well informed about colorectal cancer by doctors truly expert in the care of patients with this condition. Your family doctor, above all, will know to whom you should be referred and can act as a valuable second opinion and sounding-board. There is a lot to be told and even more to come to grips with. The knowledge that your care is in the hands of experts—combined with the support of family and friends—will see you through.

Warning signs—simple rules to follow

1. Every new case of rectal bleeding must be assessed by a doctor and, except in children, an internal rectal examination must be performed.
2. A recent change in a previously regular bowel habit that has continued for more than two weeks must be assessed by a doctor.
3. If you have a first degree relative (parent, sister, brother, or child) who has had colorectal cancer you must undergo regular colonoscopies for early detection or prevention.

Crohn's disease

Crohn's disease is an inflammatory condition that can affect almost any part of the gastrointestinal tract—from the mouth down to the anus! This can appear for the first time at almost any age from early childhood to late old-age. Once it does appear, however, it tends to remain as an ongoing source of trouble, always threatening to flare up or recur, often requiring medication to keep it under control and, not infrequently, needing surgery when it gets out of control.

The inflammation in Crohn's disease causes deep ulceration to occur at the points that are affected. This may cause diarrhoea, internal bleeding, intestinal obstruction due to stricture formation, abscesses, perforation, and erosion into surrounding structures such as the bladder, large intestine, and vagina. Active Crohn's disease may also cause significant weight loss and malnutrition.

Crohn's disease is not a cancer. But it can cause very serious illness and does tend to be a life-long problem. Those of you who have Crohn's disease can attest to the trials and tribulations of living with its complications! It is a complex disease and it cannot possibly be covered completely in this brief book. Just the same I will attempt to explain what causes Crohn's disease and how we can treat it.

What causes Crohn's disease?

We don't know! Despite our advanced understanding of so many medical conditions and despite the most up-to-date technology available for research, we still do not know exactly what causes Crohn's disease. The 'evidence' we do have is conflicting and there have been many different theories proposed over the last sixty years.

In general we believe that:

1. Affected individuals are likely to have an inbuilt genetic susceptibility to develop Crohn's disease at some stage in their lives. This might explain the frequent clustering of Crohn's disease in certain families.

2. Exposure to an organism—bacteria or a 'bug'—may provoke the inflammatory response in these susceptible individuals. This might explain the resemblance of the microscopic features of Crohn's inflammation to the changes also seen in certain infections like tuberculosis. It might also explain the fact that the anti-tuberculous antibiotics can be used to treat some cases of Crohn's disease.

3. Exposure to other environmental agents may also trigger Crohn's disease. This might be something in the food we eat, such as gluten, lactose, preservatives, and other chemicals. Some centres have described the successful treatment of patients with Crohn's disease by eliminating one or all of these elements from their diet.

Equally, cigarette smoke appears to aggravate or pro-voke Crohn's disease. Smoke may be swallowed and chemicals contained within the smoke may be responsible for triggering Crohn's inflammation.

4. It is the body's own immune system that reacts to these triggers to generate the visible changes of Crohn's disease. The immune system reaction results in 'clogging' of the tiniest blood vessels in the wall of the affected segments of intestine. This effectively deprives the intestine at these points of its normal blood supply. The involvement of the immune system in causing Crohn's disease explains why drugs that suppress the body's usual immune responses—steroids, for example—are the mainstay of drug treatment for Crohn's disease.

The long and the short of it is that we do not yet know who is going to get Crohn's disease, what exactly pro-vokes it in these individuals, and, most importantly, what they might do to prevent it from being provoked. We do know that it can run in families and that smoking, in particular, aggravates it. We must patiently wait for medical research to fill in the very large blanks in our current knowledge.

How is Crohn's disease treated?

The correct treatment of Crohn's disease depends of course on which part or parts of the gastrointestinal tract it involves and on what problems it is causing at those points. No two cases of Crohn's disease are ever exactly alike and treatment must always be tailored to suit the unique combination of which bits are affected and how badly for every individual.

Some general guidelines follow. But these are only guidelines; your own doctor will be in the best position to advise you on the correct treatment for your own situation.

1. Stop smoking

Now I am not a rabid anti-smoker! For the most part, smokers inflict harm only upon themselves. It could be argued that it is within their rights to do so. But make no mistake; if you have Crohn's disease, smoking is likely to make it worse, likely to reduce the effectiveness of drug treatment, and likely to speed up the reappearance of Crohn's disease after surgical removal. Put simply, Crohn's disease and smoking just do not mix!

2. Anti-inflammatory drugs

These include the generally mild non-steroidal agents (sulfasalazine, mesalazine, and olsalazine) as well as the more potent agents (prednisolone, budesonide, and hydrocortisone). Both groups reduce the body's overall inflammatory response and may be useful in bringing flare-ups of Crohn's disease under control.

Steroid agents also interfere with the body's immune response and tend, therefore, to be more powerful. Not surprisingly, they also tend to have many more side-effects, especially when used at high doses and for lengthy periods. Your doctor can explain the possible side-effects of steroid treatment and weigh these against the likely benefits of controlling your Crohn's disease. The balance between benefits and side-effects of drug treatment in Crohn's disease is always a critical issue.

3. Immunosuppressant drugs

These include Azathioprine (Imuran), 6-mercaptopurine, and the newer 'immunomodulating' agents such as cyclosporin and infliximab. Each of these drugs has a role in controlling the symptoms of Crohn's disease. But by interfering with the body's overall immune system, each can also have potentially serious side-effects. They need to be monitored closely by a doctor familiar with their side-effects and experienced in evaluating whether or not they are actually doing any good.

4. Surgery

The types of surgery required in Crohn's disease range from simple drainage of a perianal abscess to extensive intestinal resection, even with construction of a colostomy or ileostomy (stoma or bag). Generally, surgeons are reluctant to recommend resection of intestine since there is a strong tendency for Crohn's disease to recur even after removal of all the visibly affected segments of intestine.

But if there is major haemorrhage, obvious blockage, abscess formation, or erosion into surrounding structures, (bladder, vagina, etc.) surgery may be unavoidable. Likewise, if the side-effects of medical treatment become too serious, surgery may be the only way to allow you to escape the effects of these drugs.

Who should look after people with Crohn's disease?

The best management of your Crohn's disease will often involve a wide range of people:

(1) a specialist gastroenterologist to supervise the drug treatment and monitor your response;

(2) a colorectal surgeon to advise on the timing and nature of surgery;

(3) a dietician to ensure best nutrition and bowel habit;

(4) an enterostomal therapist to discuss issues pertaining to an ileostomy or colostomy;

(5) a family doctor, above all, to guide your overall treatment and to provide support and advice to you and your family.

Crohn's disease is, at times, a disabling condition. It can dominate your life, sometimes over many years. The advice of a trusted family doctor and specialists expert in its management are essential. And don't despair! Although the cause of Crohn's disease remains largely a mystery, research into this frustrating disease continues worldwide. Improved treatment, if not complete cure, will hopefully follow in time.

Ulcerative colitis

Like Crohn's disease, ulcerative colitis is an inflammatory disease affecting the intestines. It is not cancer. And like

Crohn's disease, we still know far too little about how and why it occurs.

But there is one very big difference between ulcerative colitis and Crohn's disease: ulcerative colitis only ever attacks the large intestine, never the small intestine and never the anus.

Of course, ulcerative colitis differs from Crohn's disease in other ways as well. The inflammation of ulcerative colitis mainly affects the superficial layers of the bowel wall whereas it extends more deeply through all layers in Crohn's disease (see Fig. 9.2). The inflammation in ulcerative colitis nearly always starts in the lowest part of the rectum and progresses upwards into the sigmoid colon, descending colon, and higher still as it becomes more extensive. In Crohn's disease, however, the inflammation generally occurs in one—or many—discrete segments of intestine leaving the intervening lengths essentially unaffected.

But the really critical difference between the two conditions is that ulcerative colitis, however severe, only affects the large intestine—the rectum and the colon. This means that it usually presents in a consistent way with varying degrees of rectal bleeding and diarrhoea. It also means that, if all other treatment fails, surgical removal of the large intestine will cure the problem forever. In Crohn's disease, there is always the possibility that the inflammation will reappear in the future, even after the most extensive resection.

So how does ulcerative colitis present?

This depends, of course, on the extent of involvement—how much of the rectum and colon is affected—as well as the severity of the inflammatory process itself.

Proctitis

In its mildest form, ulcerative colitis may be confined to the rectum. This is often called **proctitis**. It causes both bleeding and the passage of mucus with bowel actions because the inflamed rectal surface layer becomes easily broken and even frankly ulcerated. It also causes people to experience a sense of urgency accompanying their bowel actions as the inflamed rectum becomes swollen and less distensible.

Sometimes, people with proctitis visit the toilet many times a day to open their bowels only to pass a little blood, mucus, and gas. Yet their bowel motions remain normally formed and not truly loose because it is only the rectum—the final storage place for faeces—that is inflamed and irritable.

Proctitis of this sort can wax and wane over many years. During flare-ups, bleeding, mucus, and urgency may become bad enough to warrant treatment. Such treatment usually involves taking anti-inflammatory tablets (Sulfasalazine, Mesalazine) combined with anti-inflammatory steroid enemas or suppositories (Prednisolone). Because the inflammation is confined to the rectum, it is not usually necessary or appropriate to give these steroids by mouth. When taken by mouth, steroids such as Prednisolone can have significant long-term side-effects (see 3(a), below).

For people whose proctitis comes and goes over many years, a continuous course of Sulfasalazine or Mesalazine may help prevent flare-ups. No one knows better than these individuals themselves when their proctitis is flaring up and when, therefore, steroid enemas and suppositories should be reintroduced to keep the symptoms under control.

Fortunately, for the majority of people with proctitis, their inflammation remains confined to the rectum. They manage throughout their lives with their flare-ups, with their intermittent course of tablets, enemas, and suppositories and with occasional medical check-ups when things don't settle to their satisfaction. Only a small percentage ever go on to develop more extensive ulcerative colitis.

Fulminant (rapidly progressive) colitis

At the other end of the spectrum is a group of individuals who, over a period of just a few weeks, go from good health to rapidly progressive bloody diarrhoea, due to

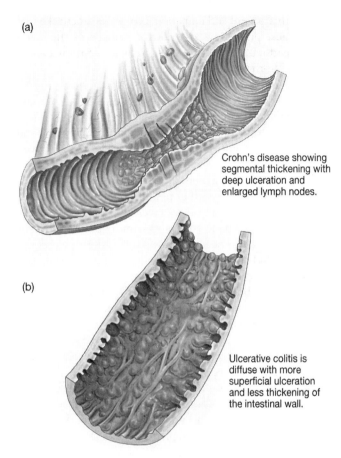

(a)

Crohn's disease showing
segmental thickening with
deep ulceration and
enlarged lymph nodes.

(b)

Ulcerative colitis is
diffuse with more
superficial ulceration
and less thickening of
the intestinal wall.

Fig. 9.2 Comparison of the inflammation and ulceration
associated with (a) Crohn's disease and (b) ulcerative colitis.

severe and extensive inflammation affecting most of the
surface of their rectum and colon. Not only do these
individuals lose enough blood to cause anaemia and to
need blood transfusions; they also lose body fluid and
protein. This can lead to dehydration and to what is, in
effect, malnutrition.

If this severe inflammation progresses unchecked, it can cause dramatic and sudden distension of the colon with perforation. In turn, this produces peritonitis and a rapid, life-threatening deterioration.

Clearly, ulcerative colitis in this severe form represents a dangerous situation. Immediate admission to hospital under the care of an expert physician or surgeon is essential. Rest in bed, attention to adequate nutrition, and high doses of anti-inflammatory steroids, usually given intravenously, are all vital elements of the treatment of these seriously ill patients. Sometimes—often as a desperate last measure—other powerful, immunosuppressant drugs such as cyclosporin are given.

Failure to respond to this programme of treatment results in worsening diarrhoea and blood loss, increasing abdominal pain and distension, and, finally, a rising pulse rate and falling blood pressure. In medical terms, this grave condition is known as **shock**. Uncorrected, death will soon follow.

Clearly, drastic action must be taken to control this situation. Even better, action should be instituted before peritonitis and shock have been allowed to develop. In these individuals, the 'drastic action' that is required is a major abdominal operation to remove most of the large intestine, preserving only the rectum. At this stage the small intestine is brought out onto the surface of the abdomen as an ileostomy and the upper end of the rectum is sealed with sutures or staples (Figure 9.3).

Only after the seriously inflamed colon has been removed is recovery possible for these individuals. Once the early post-operative phase has been successfully negotiated, there is a gradual return to normal health and nutrition. In good health, and no longer taking steroids and immunosuppressant medications, further surgery to remove the diseased rectum can be contemplated at leisure.

Chronic ulcerative colitis

Fortunately, many first attacks of ulcerative colitis are not quite as severe as in this description! What is more,

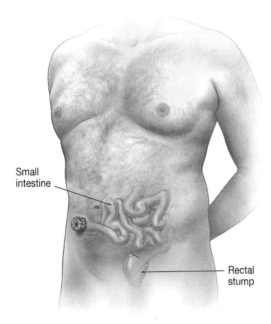

Small intestine

Rectal stump

Fig. 9.3 Total colectomy for severe colitis with closing over of the rectum and construction of an ileostomy.

most severe flare-ups do respond to the rest, attention to nutrition, and steroid therapy outlined above. In fact, many people with ulcerative colitis manage their moderately extensive and moderately severe disease at home and at work under the supervision of a specialist gastroenterologist and their family doctor for man years. These people also experience flare-ups and remissions. Their need for medication—oral Sulfasalazine, Mesalazine, Prednisolone, Budesonide, and enemas such as Prednisolone and Mesalazine taken alone or in combination—vary from week to week and from month to month.

This situation can continue for many years, even for life. For a number of reasons, however, it may be advisable for individuals to abandon their long-standing medication in favour of surgery and a permanent cure.

The side-effects of oral steroids

The long-term use of oral Prednisolone may be associated with a wide variety of adverse side-effects. There is a tendency towards fluid retention and high blood pressure. There may also be weight gain and an altered distribution of body fat, producing a round, 'moon' face and increased abdominal girth. Thinning of bones (osteoporosis) and diabetes are also possible consequences. In short, for many people, this medication causes more trouble than the ulcerative colitis itself! Better, then, to remove the disease and return to a drug-free existence.

Chronic ill-health

As they say, there is a big difference between winning and just losing slowly! Many people 'manage' while taking the medication but never really thrive. They remain continually fatigued, held back both socially and in their careers, and restricted by a chronically unsatisfactory bowel habit. Life becomes an exercise in endurance, a mere existence rather than a full and rewarding experience. Complete eradication of their disease by surgery becomes the only way for these individuals to fulfil their potential and gain the most out of life.

Repeated flare-ups

Despite their generally steady state, people with chronic ulcerative colitis often continue to experience intermittent exacerbations of their inflammation. Flare-ups may be associated with repeated admissions to hospital, recurrent blood transfusions, loss of weight, time off work, and time away from home and family. And with each exacerbation comes the prospect of urgent surgery. The unpredictability and disruption associated with these fluctuations can make life difficult to control. Only surgery can put these people back in the driver's seat.

The risk of cancer

If people with ulcerative colitis don't already have enough to contend with, they must also confront the prospect that long-standing inflammation of the colon and rectum predisposes them to colorectal cancer! This also applies to Crohn's disease affecting both the colon and rectum over many years. What is more, the tumour that arises in ulcerative colitis doesn't always start off as a visible polyp, making it even more difficult to predict which of these people will or will not develop cancer. Even when feeling well and even when taking little or no medication for their colitis, people who have had long-standing ulcerative colitis must have regular (annual) colonoscopies. Biopsies must be taken from random points throughout the colon and rectum. If these biopsies show the earliest signs of a change towards cancer—we call these changes dysplasia— or if adenomatous polyps develop in the large intestine, complete surgical removal of the colon or rectum becomes an essential means of preventing colorectal cancer.

Curative surgery

By removing the entire colon and rectum, ulcerative colitis can be cured. Although it is tempting to remove only that segment of intestine obviously affected at the time of surgery, active disease is always likely to develop in any segment of colon preserved. This will result in the need for more medical treatment, repeated colonoscopies for surveillance, the ongoing risk of developing colorectal cancer, and almost inevitably, further major surgery. Unfortunately, surgery for ulcerative colitis really does mean total resection of the colon and rectum.

Once the entire colon and rectum has been resected, the small intestine can be brought out onto the abdominal wall as an ileostomy. If the anal canal is also removed at surgery, this ileostomy will be permanent. The ulcerative colitis has been eradicated forever but these individuals will have to adjust to the rest of their lives with a stoma.

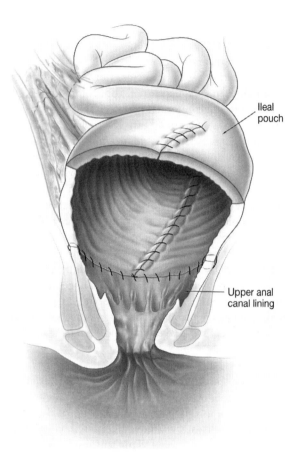

Ileal
pouch

Upper anal
canal lining

Fig. 9.4 Ileal pouch procedure. The last thirty to forty centimetres of the terminal ileum has been fashioned into a pouch and the pouch joined onto the anal canal. The muscles of the pelvic floor and the anal sphincter have been preserved.

Yet ulcerative colitis does not actually involve the anus itself and it certainly does not involve the anal sphincter muscles. This makes it possible to retain the anal canal and still 'cure' the patient of their colitis. The small intestine is rejoined onto the upper part of the anal canal restoring intestinal continuity and permitting the anus to serve its intended purpose!

Trial and error has taught us that joining the end of the terminal ileum directly onto the upper anal canal results in unmanageable diarrhoea. But by fashioning a reservoir or pouch using the last thirty to forty centimetres (twelve to sixteen inches) of the ileum and by then joining this pouch onto the anal canal, quite satisfactory bowel function can generally be achieved. This is often called the **ileal pouch** or **J-pouch procedure**.

It would be quite misleading to suggest that bowel function after the pouch procedure is always satisfactory and equally wrong to imply that this complex and often demanding operation carries no added risks or difficulties. The decision to proceed to the pouch procedure—rather than accept a permanent ileostomy—should only be made after a thorough explanation from a colorectal surgeon. Few other specialists are as well informed about the subtleties and complexities of pouch surgery and about what life is like after pouch construction.

The pouch procedure is appealing because it avoids a permanent ileostomy. But this appeal should not get in the way of a detailed analysis of the alternatives. Consider them carefully!

10
Pregnancy, birth, bowels, and bottoms

Carrying and then giving birth to a baby can place enormous strain on even the fittest and best-prepared pelvic floor. No amount of pelvic floor exercises or aqua-aerobics can guarantee freedom from anal, perianal, and pelvic floor problems either during the many months of pregnancy or in the critical hours of the delivery itself.

The female undercarriage—properly called the **perineum**—is rarely unaffected by pregnancy and vaginal delivery. Most of these problems are transient nuisances only. Some, however, are ongoing sources of discomfort and pain. And, occasionally, problems provoked by a difficult or even traumatic vaginal delivery can cause lasting distress and disability.

Even in the current era of antenatal classes, pelvic floor exercises, and informed consent, surprisingly little information about 'what really happens' to the female perineum in the course of pregnancy and delivery is available. Like so many other aspects of the information provided to women about anything from conception to parenthood, the information about their perineum and perianal region that is available tends to paint a rosy, sanitized picture as if the truth were too terrible to confront!

The emphasis on the 'natural' aspects of delivery, in particular, may be reassuring at the time. But there are many women, sadder but wiser, who feel betrayed by the unfulfilled expectations of a rapid return to their pre-pregnancy state.

The aim of this chapter is not, of course, to do the complete reverse and create fear and anxiety in expectant mothers and an avalanche of requests for planned Caesarean deliveries! The aim is to explain what can and does happen to the pelvic floor, how it can and does affect the anus and perianal region, what to look out for, and how to sort it out.

Pregnancy

Overall, pregnancy itself doesn't have a big impact on bowel function or on the perianal region until the final months. Some women, already prone to constipation by virtue of a naturally slow colonic transit (see Chapter 4; Chapter 7 on colonic inertia), do experience a further slowing of bowel transit during pregnancy. This can lead to quite troublesome constipation and, with it, undue straining at stool. This, in turn, can create anal and perianal problems such as haemorrhoids and external anal thromboses (see Chapter 5).

As your pregnancy enters its last four to six weeks and your ever-growing baby starts to press down into your pelvis, anal problems begin in earnest. With your baby's head or other body parts now occupying your pelvis, the external pressure on your rectum can give the feeling of a need to evacuate when there isn't much to do! Equally, you may leave the toilet after a bowel action with the feeling that there are still more faeces to pass. As a result, straining to evacuate your rectum commonly develops.

Add to this the inevitable congestion of haemorrhoidal and perianal blood vessels, whose normal channels of drainage are now compressed by your swollen uterus, and the scene is set for engorgement and turbulence within these blood vessels. This produces haemorrhoidal bleeding and prolapse, and—more commonly still—external anal and haemorrhoidal thromboses.

In the awkward, uncomfortable last weeks of pregnancy, sudden and painful perianal thrombosis or uncomfortable prolapse of piles can leave you feeling quite miserable.

At this late stage of pregnancy, however, there is little that can—or should—be done. If minor thromboses can be dealt with under local anaesthetic then this is not unreasonable. For more extensive thromboses as well as for more typical haemorrhoidal prolapse and bleeding, patience and sympathy are necessary! Luckily, you shouldn't have long to wait!

Delivery

Those of you who proceed to give birth by Caesarean section are much less likely to experience the adverse perianal, anal, and perineal consequences of giving birth by vaginal delivery. Common to both these modes of delivery, however, is the effect upon your bowels not only of a degree of a pain, but also of the effects of the painkillers taken for that pain. Add to this the stress of your new arrival, worries about breast-feeding, the reaction of other family members, and the prospect of going home to an absolute nightmare of neglected home duties! All these factors can interfere with normal bowel function, usually in favour of constipation. In this manner, any woman who has just given birth is prone to problems with her tail end!

But, to be fair, it is vaginal delivery that tends to cause the most trouble. You don't need to be Isaac Newton to appreciate the forces at play in getting a solid ball the size of a canteloupe melon (your baby's head) through what was previously only about a four-centimetre diameter opening in the pelvic floor muscles! Getting that same head out of the external vaginal opening itself hardly bears thinking about. Notwithstanding the natural elasticity of your body's tissues, enhanced in late pregnancy by an increase in the levels of hormones that promote such elasticity, normal vaginal delivery is always going to be a tight fit.

The degree of stretch encountered by the tissues of your pelvic floor, vagina, and perineal skin is considerable. Once stretched, the tissues generally recover tone over time but this process may take six weeks or more. Disappointingly, full recovery does not always occur. Ask any woman who has delivered vaginally and the answer will generally be that 'things are never the same again'. This is not to say that they are always worse or that many of the changes woman notice are not, in fact, quite subtle. But it is pointless to pretend that badly over-stretched tissues always return to normal. They often do not.

The pudendal nerves

One of the structures that gets stretched along the way is the pudendal nerve, which runs on the surface of the pelvic floor muscles, one on each side. Overstretching of these nerves causes a temporary reduction of nerve supply to the muscles of the pelvic floor and to the external anal sphincter muscle. Since we rely on these muscles to provide extra 'grip' when the urge to have our bowels open arrives, stretch injury to the pudendal nerves at the time of vaginal delivery can cause problems with urgency and incontinence of faeces. Whilst this also recovers over time, recovery is not always complete.

In fact, some degree of permanent stretch injury to the pudendal nerves, as well as to the tissues of the vagina and pelvic floor, should be regarded as part and parcel of normal vaginal delivery and not at all as a horrendous complication of the process.

Tears

Of course, your body's tissues will not continue to stretch indefinitely but may reach a breaking point along the way. If the pelvic floor won't stretch or the bony pelvis cannot accommodate your baby's head, normal vaginal delivery cannot proceed. This can be an urgent situation and your obstetrician or midwife will recognize the need to proceed to an alternative means of delivery: vacuum, forceps, or Caesarean.

But if the pelvic floor allows your baby through only to find that the vaginal outlet will not, then its stretching may give way to tearing. A carefully timed surgical cut of the perineal skin heading into the vagina itself can effectively enlarge the vaginal outlet and avoid an untidy skin tear. This cut is correctly called an **episiotomy**.

Even with an episiotomy, however, some unplanned tearing of the skin can still occur. Both planned episiotomies and unplanned tears are sutured back in place after your baby has been delivered. The swelling and pain associated with the sutures can interfere with normal bowel and bladder function for a number of days.

A more important and serious tear is one that involves the anal sphincter muscle. As I have already explained (see Chapter 3), the anus is surrounded by two cylinders of muscle: the internal and external sphincter muscles. These are vital components of the mechanism that gives us continence over gas and faeces. The front part of the sphincter ring lies between the anus and vagina. As your baby's head reaches a point just a few centimetres away from the external vaginal opening, it makes contact with the upper edge of the front part of the sphincter ring. Where there is plenty of room in your pelvis and the descent of your baby's head occurs in a steady and controlled fashion, the anal sphincter mechanism gets pushed backwards and out of harm's way.

In other circumstances—not enough room or not enough time—the force of your baby's head passing down and out can compress and split the upper end of the anal sphincter mechanism, effectively leaving the front part of the sphincter cylinder shortened (Figure 10.1). This is a surprisingly frequent occurrence (perhaps in as many as one third of vaginal deliveries), but it causes very little in the way of incontinence. It is probably yet another 'normal' aspect of vaginal delivery and not, in itself, a cause of significant trouble.

Only rarely (perhaps only 1–2 per cent of cases), tearing of the front part of the anal sphincter mechanism extends down all or very nearly all of the length of the sphincter muscle. With little or none of the sphincter intact throughout its full circumference, there is now noticeable loss of control over gas and faeces.

Often in such cases there is also tearing of the vaginal lining as well. Your obstetrician or midwife will recognize the sphincter injury and take steps to repair it. If this repair is unsuccessful, or if the original tear goes unrecognized, an ongoing disturbance of continence is likely. There is no mistaking anal sphincter tear after vaginal delivery. It causes an immediate and quite definite loss of anal control.

At the extreme end of the spectrum of anal sphincter injury is a complete tear of the back wall of the vagina, anal sphincter muscle, and lining of the anal canal and lower rectum. This, too, can be repaired at the time of delivery, although breakdown of any of the suture lines

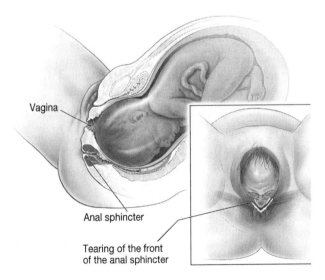

Fig. 10.1 Tearing of the anal sphincter muscles by traumatic passage of the fetal head during vaginal delivery.

might then result not only in a degree of incontinence, but also in formation of a false passage from the anus and rectum into the vagina. This rare complication of vaginal delivery is called a recto-vaginal fistula. It causes gas and faeces to be passed, without control, through the vagina. This is an obviously distressing, though generally rare, occurrence. It can be corrected surgically but requires the attention of a surgeon expert in the care of this condition.

Summary: anal and perianal complications of pregnancy and childbirth

External anal thrombosis

These are sudden, painful perianal swellings due to thrombosis (clotting) within the blood vessels that run in the tissue just beneath the skin of the lowest part of the anal canal. This is an extremely common condition, often incorrectly called 'thrombosed haemorrhoids'. Although very painful at first, they always subside of their own accord and should not, as a general rule, be operated upon in the event of a recent vaginal delivery. Getting your bowels open after delivery is hard enough without having also to contend with one or more raw painful perianal wounds. Ice packs, soothing lotions, analgesics, and plenty of compassion are in order. And remember: don't let anyone attempt to push these painful lumps back up or anywhere else! It never helps and it can be very painful.

Haemorrhoids

Bleeding, prolapse, and even thrombosis of true haemorrhoids can also complicate late pregnancy and delivery. Since the obvious aggravating factor has been taken away (delivered, more accurately) there is every prospect that the haemorrhoids themselves will also resolve of their own accord. In any event, the immediate post-delivery period is an awful time to have to undergo haemorrhoidectomy. Again, a patient approach to your haemorrhoids is preferred. If your haemorrhoids continue to bleed and prolapse three months after delivery then you may reconsider the sorts of treatments already outlined in Chapter 5.

Anal fissure

Anal thrombosis and haemorrhoids tend to clear up very quickly in the week or two after giving birth. Lingering anal pain and bleeding should immediately suggest an anal fissure. But such is the general level of ignorance about common anal complaints (and such is the belief amongst new mothers that a painful undercarriage is to be expected!) that symptoms can drag on for months before attention is sought.

Anal fissure is discussed in detail in Chapter 5. In short, if you have come to dread having a bowel action because of pain, you have an anal fissure, not a haemorrhoid, and relief may be readily available, either with local cream or, occasionally, minor anal surgery.

Incontinence

Incontinence of faeces is a humiliating experience. For this to occur in an otherwise fit young woman, quite without warning and at a time when she had expected to be celebrating a major lifetime milestone, can be utterly devastating. Added to the usual stresses of life with a tiny baby, incontinence of faeces may be more than enough to precipitate depression.

The good news is that incontinence due to an anal sphincter tear does respond well to surgical repair. This is best left for at least three to four months after delivery to allow the swollen tissues to recover and fibrous scarring to 'mature'. The fibrous scar tissue holds sutures well and is definitely helpful at the time of surgical repair.

If you require anal sphincter repair you should be assessed and treated by a surgeon expert in this procedure.

Your family doctor or obstetrician will be able to direct
you to an appropriate specialist.

Pelvic floor weakness

The after-effects of 'the big stretch' are numerous. The
vagina is often more capacious, altering sensation for both
participants once sex restarts. Many of these effects are
not really noticed until later in life, perhaps due to the
combined effect of several vaginal deliveries and middle
age. The various forms of vaginal prolapse are good exam-
ples of the weakening of the normal pelvic supporting tissues, which develops in later life largely as a result of the
traumas of vaginal delivery.

Similarly, the combined effect of vaginal delivery on
the pudendal nerves might also contribute, in later life, to
a degree of sphincter weakness sufficient to cause incontinence. Big babies, long labours, and the use of instruments (forceps and vacuum) all increase the likelihood
of significant pudendal nerve stretch injury. When the
sphincter muscle is intact but weakened by nerve injury,
surgical repair is much less likely to help. Attention to
other, equally important, factors such as firming the stool
consistency (see Chapter 3) is generally more rewarding
than surgery. Again, the assessment and advice of a surgeon expert in the care of anal incontinence is essential.

Common problems seen during pregnancy and after childbirth

(1) haemorrhoidal bleeding and prolapse;

(2) painful external anal and haemorrhoidal thromboses;

(3) chronic anal fissure;

(4) reduced control over gas and faeces.

11
Colonic irrigation and other quackery

As already discussed, many complaints arising from bowel and bottom are troublesome but not life-threatening. A nuisance, a bother, an irritation, but not too serious.

And many of these complaints come and go of their own accord whether or not we find out what caused them and whether or not we actually do anything about them. What a perfect arena this is, then, for the well-meaning opportunist or for the charlatan with a view to a quick profit! Regardless of the efficacy of their new 'wonder' treatment, the health problem itself is likely to resolve of its own accord sooner or later. And even if it doesn't, the problem is never likely to be too serious so it's a case of 'no harm done'.

What a strange and unprincipled way to deliver any sort of service, let alone the care of another human being. Science and the 'medical model' do not have all the answers for a long and healthy life. But illogical notions disguised in semi-scientific language cannot possibly fill in the gaps.

There are two main areas of colonic quackery. One, which I have already discussed in Chapter 5 on haemorrhoids, relates to the various treatments available for minor perianal symptoms such as itching, pain, and bleeding. All these symptoms are generally lumped together as 'haemorrhoids'.

Such treatments prey on people's powerful reluctance to discuss anorectal symptoms with anyone at all and their preference for grabbing the treatment off the pharmacy shelf, then escaping with it as quickly and as anonymously as possible. The fundamentals of best treatment are ignored, and considerable and unnecessary expense is incurred. For those of you with these anal and perianal complaints, I urge you to save your money, read Chapter 5, and sort it out properly.

The other area in which quackery has taken a firm hold is in the area of colonic irrigation. In this treatment, a tube is inserted into the rectum through the anal canal, then varying volumes and types of fluid are instilled. This is, of course, nothing more than a large enema. The lining of the large bowel cannot absorb much more than a little bit of water and the tiniest amount of salt. Any fluid that is administered in the process of colonic irrigation simply passes back out of the anal canal, taking some of the faeces in the colon out with it.

The basic notion behind colonic irrigation is that faeces contain 'toxins' that are poisonous to the body system as a whole. It is true that at least half the weight of normal human faeces is made up of bacteria. If faeces were to find their way outside the intestine—into the general abdominal cavity, where they would cause peritonitis, or into the bloodstream, where they would cause septicaemia—this would clearly be a serious situation. So I suppose it is true that the content of faeces is toxic but only if it finds its way into the wrong place.

But the simple truth is that there is no safer place for faeces to be than inside the intestines themselves. The intestines are ideally designed to extract from bowel content the fluid and the nutrients that the body needs. A healthy intestine is able to contain these 'toxins' within the bowel where they belong. Flushing out otherwise normal faeces is completely illogical and potentially harmful.

On the other hand, if the intestine is diseased—and particularly if there is ulceration of the surface of the intestine—there is the very real prospect that the bacterial toxins present within faeces may be absorbed into the bloodstream or may contaminate the abdominal cavity in the event of intestinal perforation. If there is an underlying disease affecting the large intestine, colonic irrigation is exceedingly dangerous because the instillation of a large volume of fluid increases the pressure within the large bowel. This may be just enough to tip the balance in favour of perforation, which really will cause the release of toxins into the system!

I'm afraid to say that there really is no justification whatsoever for performing colonic irrigation except in the circumstance where it is used as an enema for people with problematic constipation. Even in this situation, it is only advisable as a one-off treatment; a sensible regime of powerful laxatives, as outlined in Chapter 4, is a much more sensible and sustainable long-term treatment for people with such severe constipation.

There are many, many people who make their living from caring for sick people or people with troublesome symptoms. This includes medical doctors, of course. A lot of these treatments—including those provided by doctors—are expensive and potentially harmful. So it is fair to say that the treatments prescribed by doctors—and I include myself in this group—are neither always successful nor by any means cheap.

This is, however, no reason to abandon scientific fact, let alone common sense, in trying to control your symptoms and illnesses. When it comes to problems relating to bowels and bottoms, the vast majority of people are extremely vulnerable to the quasi-medical, pseudo-scientific nonsense so often directed at the treatment of perianal symptoms and best exemplified by the whole colonic irrigation racket. I urge you to read the explanations provided in this book, implement the recommendations that are contained within it, and seek assistance and guidance from your family doctor or an appropriate specialist if you do not meet with success.

Above all, don't abandon plain common sense. And don't allow any unqualified individual to stick anything at all up your bottom end!

Recap: When bowel motions get too soft

There is no doubt that constipation because of slow colonic transit and bowel motions that have become too hard is a common problem. Yet, we have never been better informed about the benefits of increasing our dietary fibre and have been well and truly brainwashed into believing that we must all strive to achieve a consistently soft bowel motion.

For the record, dietary fibre does play an important role in providing us with essential vitamins not available from other dietary sources. What is more, fibre can help lower blood cholesterol levels and appears to have a protective effect against the development of bowel cancer and, probably, breast cancer. So it's true: fibre *is* good for you. But where is it written that if a little of something is good for you, then a whole bucketful is necessarily better? And why should it be true that if more fibre *is* good for some of us, then it just *has* to be good for everyone else too?

As I've pointed out in almost every chapter of this book, many people suffer the consequences of having too soft a bowel motion and of having to make too many visits to the toilet to have their bowels open. The adverse consequences of too soft and frequent a bowel habit include powerful and distressing urges to pass gas or have a bowel action, even to the point of producing a humiliating episode of incontinence. Less dramatic (but equally upsetting) can be difficulties in completing a bowel action. This may result in prolonged straining at stool, lengthy attempts to 'clean up' after a bowel action, soiling or incontinence without warning immediately after a bowel action, and perianal itching and burning discomfort. If you have any of these symptoms and your motions are soft or frequent, you may well benefit from the pursuit of a more solid stool consistency.

What can you do to make your bowel motions more solid?

The best and most obvious way for any of us to make our motions more solid is by changing our diet to reduce the intake of foods and drinks that make us softer and to replace them with others that do not. The six main areas to concentrate on are:

1. *Vegetables.* All vegetables tend to make our motions softer and more frequent and tend to make us more gassy. Beans, broccoli, Brussels sprouts, cabbages, capsicums, corn, and onions are the vegetables with the most potent action on our bowels. On the other hand, potatoes and pumpkins appear to be the least likely to make us loose and gassy.

Obviously, vegetables form an important part of our diet and provide essential vitamins that cannot be readily obtained from other sources. But, if taken in large amounts, vegetables are likely to be a major cause of a bowel motion that is too soft.

2. *Fruit.* Again, all fruit tends to make us softer and more frequent. This is particularly so of stone fruit (apricots, grapes, peaches, and plums) and, not surprisingly, the various dried fruits (this includes prunes and sultanas). Bananas, on the other hand, tend not to have a major impact on bowel habit. People who eat large amounts of fruit—particularly stone fruit during summer time—are likely to suffer the consequences!

3. *Other sources of fibre.* These days we are constantly reminded of the important health benefits of dietary fibre. Many people take fibre supplements such as natural bran, psyllium husks or commercially available preparations

such as Fybogel, Metamucil, and Granocol (to name but a few). Most breakfast cereals also contain added bran and much of the bread we eat is impregnated with grains, bran, and other fibre supplements.

We really are living in 'high fibre times'. It can be difficult to find a decent piece of white bread, and traditionally low fibre food such as white rice and pasta are often served with sauces rich in vegetables and spices.

People whose bowel motions are already too soft rarely benefit from the intake of extra dietary fibre. Not only does this tend to make them softer but it often makes them even more gassy and uncomfortable. A simple low fibre breakfast (toasted white bread, for example) is often a highly effective first step in achieving a more solid stool consistency.

4. *Spices*. Almost everybody is familiar with the potent effect that spices such as chilli and food such as curry can have on our bowel habit. Most people are not, however, quite so familiar with the fact that cinnamon, garlic, and nutmeg may also have such an effect. Garlic, in particular, forms an important component of the daily diet of many people in whom it may be a significant cause of too soft a bowel action. Common sense and a little bit of restraint are all that is required to minimize the effect of too much spice in our diets.

5. *Caffeine*. Caffeine is a well-known stimulant. Apart from keeping us awake it also stimulates the gastrointestinal tract and can contribute to an excessively loose bowel habit. Caffeine is present not only in coffee and tea, but also in the various colas (including diet cola). For people who consume large quantities of caffeine, the decaffeinated varieties are a sensible alternative that might help keep bowel motions a little more solid.

6. *Alcohol*. Any of us who has 'overindulged' on an occasional or regular basis will know that alcohol has a very marked effect on our bowel habits. This is especially the case with beer and, to a lesser extent, wine. The more beer

or wine that we drink the looser our motions become. Spirits are generally less active on our intestines despite their much higher concentrations of alcohol.

So what is left that can be eaten?

All dietary advice needs to be applied with a large 'serving' of common sense. Reducing the amount of these foods and drinks is not the same as cutting them out altogether! Sensible, step-wise reductions are the best way to approach these dietary recommendations. Trying to make radical changes to your diet, particularly if this means withholding foods of which you are especially fond, is unlikely to be sustainable in the long term.

There are, of course, many foods that do not have such a marked effect on our bowels. As already mentioned, bananas, potatoes, and pumpkins fit into this category. Likewise pasta, white (low fibre) bread, and white rice do not make our bowels loose. Dairy products, fish, and meat are also very gentle on our bowels. As always, it is a matter of finding the right balance between essential nutrients, taste, and the effect that diet has on our bowels.

Remember, a useful first step is to make two simple changes:

1. *Turn breakfast into a low fibre meal.* Although many people have become accustomed to having a high fibre breakfast (added bran, fruit, muesli, prunes, etc.), we generally don't attach too much gastronomic weight to breakfast. In other words, breakfast is not a meal from which we demand great taste and enjoyment. It is also our most 'solitary' meal. Unlike lunch and, in particular, dinner, we rarely make breakfast for any one else. Each of us tends to prepare our own, so changing breakfast rarely affects others! It is, therefore, a convenient meal to alter without causing too much interference or making us too miserable. So instead of all that excess fibre, how about a couple of pieces of toasted white bread?

2. *Make all the bread you eat white.* Forget the crunchy, tasty, wholemeal, multigrain, megagrain breads and rolls! Insist on old-fashioned, low-fibre, white bread.

What if diet doesn't work?

For some people dietary changes are either ineffective, impractical, (vegetarians or diabetics, for example) or simply too unpleasant to sustain. In this situation anti-diarrhoeal medication may prove effective in controlling symptoms. Some of the anti-diarrhoeal medications—a good example is codeine—do have effects on the body other than acting as a constipating agent. They may produce sedation and give pain relief but they are also addictive. They may be highly effective but they are not always the best first choice.

The anti-diarrhoeal drug loperamide (which is marketed as Imodium or Gastrostop) has a very potent effect on the bowel but is barely absorbed into the bloodstream. There have been virtually no side-effects reported other than those on the intestinal tract (nausea, bloating, constipation) and it has no tendency for the development of tolerance—the need for ever-increasing doses to produce the same effect—or addiction. It can be taken even in the long term without any fear of the body getting used to its effects.

How much loperamide should I take?

This is something that really needs to be discussed carefully with your own doctor. Because its action can be very strong, loperamide should always be started at a low dose and only gradually increased according to its effects. Ultimately, however, the individual patient is the person in the best position to determine how much and how often he or she should be taking loperamide. It certainly makes sense to put simple dietary alterations in place first before starting on loperamide in order to avoid suffering from the reverse problem, namely constipation.

Finally, remember that as your bowel motions become firmer, the urge to open your bowels will become less frequent. As a result, your usual bowel pattern is likely to change. It is extremely important that visits to the toilet to open your bowels only take place when there is a sufficiently strong urge. It is a mistake to sit on the toilet in anticipation of a bowel action or in the hope that one might be achieved when you do not have a strong natural urge to do so. As your motions become more solid, please remember not to visit the toilet to have your bowels open unless the urge is strong.

13
Visiting your doctor

The prospect of visiting a doctor to discuss a problem related to our bowels is not an inviting one. Talking about the workings of our bowels is embarrassing enough but this is made worse by uncertainty as to the correct terminology to use and by the likelihood that an internal examination is going to be performed. It's little wonder that so many people leave symptoms unreported for so long, hoping that they will go away and that the inevitable humiliation will be avoided!

A thorough medical assessment of your symptoms is almost always going to involve discussion about how often you go, how easy or difficult it is to go, the consistency and even the colour of what you pass, the presence or absence of pain, prolapse, bleeding, mucus, and itching. There will be questions about abdominal pain and distension, about a family history of bowel conditions, about the birth of your children (for women), and about any previous bottom or bowel problems and operations.

And yes, a thorough medical assessment is almost certainly going to involve having an internal rectal examination, the ultimate invasion of our privacy. I have lost count of the number of women who have told me that they find an internal rectal examination to be much more intrusive and a much more daunting prospect than the equivalent gynaecological examination!

A rectal examination is both uncomfortable and undignified but it is absolutely vital if serious conditions such as cancer are not to be missed. Imagine finally summoning up the courage to talk about your symptoms and risking all that embarrassment, and yet not coming away with the assurance that all is well!

In this book I have described the common conditions that affect our bowels and bottom end. You now have a good working knowledge—possibly better than some doctors—of what symptoms relate to which diagnosis and of how to go about getting on top of them: incontinence, constipation, anal pain, bleeding, itching, and more! You now know that many of these symptoms just have 'nuisance value' and that relief can be obtained with simple strategies and common sense.

I hope that what you have learned in this book has put you back in control of your bowels and bottom end, instead of them in control of you!

But the serious conditions—the 'dangerous creatures'—must never be ignored. Seeing your doctor to discuss your symptoms and to be examined is vitally important. Armed with the correct terminology and an understanding of the workings of your most intimate opening, you can now approach your visit to the doctor with confidence, knowing better what to expect and how to interpret the advice you receive. I wish you good luck.

Index

Entries in bold type refer to figures.

Index